LIPPINCOTT'S REVIEW SERIES

Maternal-Newborn Nursing

D1357857

LIPPINCOTT'S REVIEW SERIES

Maternal-Newborn Nursing

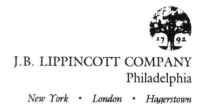

J.B. LIPPINCOTT COMPANY
Philadelphia

New York • London • Hagerstown

Sponsoring Editor: **Donna L. Hilton, RN, BSN**
Coordinating Editorial Assistant: **Susan Perry**
Project Editor: **Melissa McGrath**
Indexer: **Alexandra Nickerson**
Designer: **Doug Smock**
Production Manager: **Helen Ewan**
Production Coordinator: **Maura Murphy**
Compositor: **Pine Tree Composition, Inc.**
Printer/Binder: **R. R. Donnelley & Sons Company**
Cover Printer: **The Lehigh Press, Inc.**

6 5 4 3 2 1

Library of Congress Cataloging-in-Publication Data

Lippincott's review series : maternal-newborn nursing.
    p.   cm.
  Includes bibliographical references and index.
  ISBN 0-397-54776-5
  1. Obstetrical nursing—Examinations, questions, etc.
2. Obstetrical nursing—Outlines, syllabi, etc. I. J. B. Lippincott
Company. II. Title: Maternal-newborn nursing.
  [DNLM: 1. Obstetrical Nursing—examination questions.
2. Obstetrical Nursing—outlines. WY 18 L7652]
RG951.L57 1992
610.73'678'076—dc20
DNLM/DLC
for Library of Congress   91-29933
                                             CIP

CONTRIBUTING
AUTHORS

Nu-Vision, Inc.
Paula S. Cokingtin, RN, EdD, President
Kathy D. Robinson, RN, MSN, Vice President
Carolyn H. Brose, RN, EdD, Vice President
Linda N. Kohlman, RN, MN, Associate

Barbara Clancy, RN, EdD

Professor
Department of Maternal Health Nursing
School of Nursing
University of Kansas
Kansas City, Kansas

Mary Ann Kasper, RN, EdD

Associate Professor
Department of Maternal Health Nursing
School of Nursing
University of Kansas
Kansas City, Kansas

REVIEWERS

Helen L. Dulock, RN, MN
Assistant Professor and Project Director
Perinatal Graduate Program
Doctoral Candidate
University of California
San Franciso, California

Virginia L. Kinnick, RN, MSN, CNM
Assistant Professor
School of Nursing
University of Northern Colorado
Greeley, Colorado

Sharon A. Vinten, RNC, MSN
Professor of Nursing
Indiana University
School of Nursing
Indianapolis, Indiana

INTRODUCTION

Lippincott's Review Series is designed to help you in your study of the key subject areas in nursing. The series consists of four books, one in each core nursing subject area:

Medical-Surgical Nursing
Pediatric Nursing
Maternal-Newborn Nursing
Mental Health and Psychiatric Nursing

Each book contains a comprehensive outline content review, chapter study questions and answer keys with rationales for correct and incorrect responses, and a comprehensive examination and answer key with rationales for correct and incorrect responses.

Lippincott's Review Series was planned and developed in response to your requests for outline review books that address each major subject area and also contain a self-test mechanism. These books meet the need for comprehensive subject review books that will also assist you in identifying your strong and weak areas of knowledge. Each book is a complete source for review and self-assessment of a single core subject—all four together provide an excellent comprehensive review of entry-level nursing.

Each book is all-inclusive of the content addressed in major textbooks. The content outline review uses a consistent nursing process format throughout and addresses nursing care for well and ill clients. Also included are such necessary additional topics as developmental and life-cycle issues, health assessment, patient teaching, and other concepts including growth and development, nutrition, pharmacology, and anatomy, physiology, and pathophysiology.

You can use the books in this series in several different ways. Overall, you can use them as subject reviews to augment general study throughout your basic nursing program and as a review to prepare for the National Council Licensure Examination (NCLEX-RN). How you use each book depends on your individual needs and preferences and on whether you review each chapter systematically or concentrate only on those chapters whose subject areas are particularly problematic or challenging. You may instead choose to use the comprehensive examination as a self-assessment opportunity to evaluate your knowledge base before you review the content outline. Likewise, you can use the study questions for pre- or post-testing after study, followed by the comprehensive examination as a means of evaluating your knowledge and competencies of an entire subject area.

Regardless of how you use the books, one of the strengths of the series is the self-assessment opportunity it offers in addition to guidance in studying and reviewing content. The chapter study questions and comprehensive examination questions have been carefully developed to cover all topics in the outline review. Most importantly, each question is categorized according to the components of the National Council of State Boards of Nursing Licensing Examination (NCLEX).

- ▶ Cognitive Level: Knowledge, Comprehension, Application, or Analysis
- ▶ Client Need: Safe, Effective Care Environment (Safe Care); Physiological Integrity (Physiologic); Psychosocial Integrity (Psychosocial); and Health Promotion and Maintenance (Health Promotion)
- ▶ Phase of the Nursing Process: Assessment, Analysis (Dx), Planning, Implementation, Evaluation

For those questions not related to a client need or to a phase of the nursing process, NA (not applicable) will be used, as in questions that test knowledge of a basic science.

Unlike the NCLEX examination that tests the cumulative knowledge needed for safe practice by an entry-level nurse, these practice tests systematically evaluate the knowledge base that serves as the building block for the entire nursing educational process. In this way, you can prepare for the NCLEX examination throughout your course of study. Good study habits throughout your educational program are not only the best way to ensure on-going success, but also will prove the most beneficial way to prepare for the licensing examination.

Keep in mind that these books are not intended to replace formal learning. They cannot substitute for textbook reading, discussion with instructors, or class attendance. Every effort has been made to provide accurate and current information, but class attendance and interaction with an instructor will provide invaluable information not found in books. Used correctly, these books will help you increase understanding, improve comprehension, evaluate strengths and weaknesses in areas of knowledge, increase productive study time, and as a result help you improve your grades.

MONEY BACK GUARANTEE—Lippincott's Review Series will help you study more effectively during coursework throughout your educational program and help you prepare for quizzes and tests, including the NCLEX exam. If you buy and use any of the four volumes in Lippincott's Review Series and fail the NCLEX exam, simply send us verification of your exam results and your copy of the review book to the address below. We will promptly send you a check for our suggested list price.

Lippincott's Review Series
J. B. Lippincott Company
227 East Washington Square
Philadelphia, PA 19106-3780

CONTENTS

Introduction to Maternal-Newborn Nursing

I. Evolution of maternal-newborn nursing

  A. History of maternal-newborn care in America

      1. 1700 to 1900

        a. During this period, traditional English birth practices prevailed; the improved maternal outcome in the colonies as compared to Europe is attributed to less crowded conditions, better nutrition, and healthier women.

        b. Midwives—women experienced in attending births—were common; formal training and licensure for physicians did not occur until the mid-19th century.

        c. Thereafter, for a short while, midwifery and physician co-practice were common, with midwives being called for uncomplicated births and physicians attending complicated deliveries.

    d.   Analgesia for childbirth, introduced by Simpson in 1847, shifted childbirth from the home to the hospital by the early 20th century.

    e.   By the late 19th century, midwifery was fully absorbed into medical training as a specialty.

2.   20th century

    a.   Before 1900, less than 5% of births in the United States occurred in hospitals. As medicine became more organized, hospitals opened in large numbers, providing a centralized setting for physician practice.

    b.   The childbirth experience came to be dictated by strict hospital rules, separation of women from families during labor and birth, restriction of maternal activity during labor, transfer to delivery room for birth, and early transfer of newborn to nursery with no provisions for parent–infant contact.

    c.   Hospitals developed training programs for nurses. Nursing students provided nursing care for hospitalized patients, and graduate nurses provided in-home nursing care as employees of the families.

    d.   Legislation was passed in many states outlawing midwifery practice in the belief that hospital-based physician care was superior.

    e.   In 1918, the Maternity Center Association was founded in New York to provide care to poor women and children.

    f.   In 1925, the Frontier Nursing Service was established by Mary Breckinridge to provide care for families in remote areas of Appalachia.

    g.   By the 1970s, more than 90% of births in the United States were attended by physicians and occurred in hospitals.

B.   Influence of federal and state programs on maternal-newborn care

1.   In 1921, the Sheppard-Towner Act provided funds for state-managed maternal-child health programs.

2.   In 1930, the Sheppard-Towner Act was repealed due to political pressure exerted by organized medicine—despite evidence that mortality rates declined under these programs.

3.   In 1935, Title V of the Social Security Act was amended to provide funding for maternal-child health programs.

4.   In 1944, the Public Health Service Act brought together all existing laws affecting the public health service and provided funding for research and education of personnel needed for maternal and child health programs.

5.   In 1962, the National Institute of Child Health and Human De-

velopment was authorized. The Institute supports research and training in special health problems and needs of mothers and children, and also funds basic science research relating to human growth and development, including prenatal development.

6. In 1964, the Title V amendment to the Public Health Service Act established the Maternal and Infant Care (MIC) projects, emphasizing comprehensive prenatal and infant care in public centers.

7. In 1965, Title XIX of the Medicaid Program, MCH Services Block Grant, provided funds to facilitate access to care by pregnant women and young children.

8. In 1965, phenylketonuria testing became mandatory for all infants in the states of Illinois and Michigan, thus setting a precedent for other states.

9. In 1966, the Department of Health, Education, and Welfare (HEW) issued a policy statement on birth control, stating that the Department would support, on request, health programs making family planning information and services available.

10. In 1967, many states' Medicaid programs expanded to include care during pregnancy and child care.

11. In 1968, Head Start programs began providing educational opportunities for low-income children of preschool age.

12. In 1969, the National Center for Family Planning was established under the Health Services and Mental Health Administration, HEW, to serve as a clearing house for contraceptive information.

13. In 1973, the National Center on Child Abuse and Neglect was established in HEW's Office of Child Development to act as a clearing house for information about child abuse.

14. In 1975, the Women, Infants, and Children (WIC) program, a supplemental food program directed at providing supplemental foods and nutrition education for low-income families, was established.

15. In 1976, the Early and Periodic Screening, Diagnostic and Treatment (EPSDT) program began providing Medicaid-eligible children with regular health screening and treatment through federal funding.

16. In 1977, the Child Health Assessment Act (CHAP) extended the EPSDT program to broaden eligibility and to require that treatment be given for conditions discovered during assessment.

C. Development of nurse–midwifery in America

1. In 1932, the Maternity Center Association began training public health nurses in midwifery practice in the Lobenstein School of Nurse–Midwifery.

2. In the 1930s, the Frontier Nursing Service in Kentucky began training nurses in midwifery.

3. In 1969, the American College of Nurse–Midwives was estab-

lished as the official agency for approving educational programs and certifying graduates of these programs.

4. In 1971, the first National Certification Examination for nurse-midwives was administered; the professional desgination CNM indicates certified nurse–midwife.

5. In 1981, Congress authorized Medicaid payments for the services of certified nurse–midwives.

II. Family-centered maternal-newborn nursing

A. **Description: Safe, quality nursing care that recognizes, focuses on, and adapts to both the physical and psychosocial needs of the patient, the family, and the neonate, with emphasis on fostering family unity while maintaining physical safety.**

B. Development

1. During the early 1940s, more parents began questioning the rigid hospital rules and routines associated with labor and delivery.

2. During this period, Grantly Dick-Reed introduced the concept of childbirth preparation and participation of the father in labor and delivery.

3. Arnold Gesell supported the practice of rooming-in.

4. John Bowlby began describing the tragic effects of maternal deprivation on children.

5. St. Mary's Hospital in Evansville, Indiana, established the first Family-Centered Maternity Care Program in the late 1950s; this approach quickly spread across the nation.

C. Philosophy and features

1. The basic philosophy of family-centered maternal-newborn nursing can be summed up in the following statements:

   a. Given adequate information and professional support, the family is capable of making decisions about care during the childbearing periods.

   b. In most cases, childbirth is a normal, healthy event in the life of a family.

   c. Childbirth marks the beginning of a new set of important family relationships.

2. Important features of family-centered maternal-newborn care include:

   a. Prenatal and parent education classes

   b. Family participation in labor, birth, and the postpartum period, including attendance by the father or a support person during labor and birth, unrestricted family visitation, and sibling participation

   c. Presence of support person for complicated or cesarean birth, if possible

   d. Use of a homelike birth setting

   e. Flexible policies regarding routine procedures

          f.   Postbirth recovery without routine transfer of family

          g.   Early extended parent–neonate contact

          h.   Flexible rooming-in policy

          i.   Family involvement in special neonatal care unit, including transport of mother and neonate, if necessary

          j.   Early postbirth discharge with close follow-up

    3.   Other aspects of family-centered maternal-newborn care may include:

          a.   Nontraditional labor and birth settings (e.g., in-hospital birth centers, freestanding birth centers, single-room maternity system, home birth)

          b.   Nonviolent or gentle birth practices (e.g., Leboyer method)

III. Legal and ethical issues in maternal-newborn care

  A. **Complex ethical decision-making**

    1.   Maternal vs. fetal rights involves:

          a.   Concept of the fetus as a patient separate from the mother

          b.   Forced medical treatment of the fetus against the will of the mother

    2.   Standards of fetal viability vary widely.

  B. **Litigation and professional liability**

    1.   Critical elements of professional practice in maternity nursing include:

          a.   Thorough initial history and examination to enable the nurse to identify risk factors and institute appropriate measures

          b.   Complete and accurate documentation of patient status and care rendered, regarded as the only valid record of events from a legal standpoint

          c.   Appropriate use and interpretation of fetal monitoring

    2.   Nurses are experiencing increased exposure to litigation in obstetric care, as are physicians. (Approximately 80% of all medical malpractice cases in U.S. history have been filed since 1975; nearly 75% of all OB/GYN physicians in the United States have been sued, 30% with three or more suits filed against them.)

    3.   Joint actions against both the physician and nurse are common, especially in emergency situations in which assessments and interventions occur quickly.

    4.   The increased risk for litigation arises because the majority of lawsuits claim that the infant has sustained severe birth injury and will require long-term care, that substandard care caused the injury, and because of the frequent unavailability of physicians.

    5.   Increased litigation has resulted in increased liability insurance rates for both physicians and nurses caring for childbearing families.

IV. Nursing process in maternal-newborn care

A. Assessment

1. Nursing assessment of the patient and family includes:
   a. Completion of a nursing health history
   b. Interview and observation
   c. Measurement of vital signs and physiologic indicators
   d. Review of medical records
2. Various standardized tools (Table 1–1) can aid assessment.

B. Nursing diagnoses

TABLE 1–1.

Assessment Tools Used in Maternal-Newborn Nursing

TOOL	PURPOSE	DESCRIPTION
Maternal-Fetal Attachment Scale (parent self-report)	▶ Measures aspects of maternal attachment to fetus (A paternal version has been developed and tested.)	Contains 33 written scales focusing on differentiation of self from fetus, interaction with fetus, attribution of characteristics to fetus, giving of self, and role taking.
Apgar Scoring System	▶ Allows quick, comprehensive evaluation of neonate's immediate adaptation to birth process and extrauterine life ▶ Indicates extent to which newborn requires more vigorous management or resuscitation	Rates five components (heart rate, respiratory effort, muscle tone, reflex irritability, and color) on a scale from 0 to 2. Ratings are done at 1 and 5 minutes after birth. Scores of 0 to 3 reflect severe distress; 4 to 6 moderate distress; and 7 to 10, mild or absent distress.
Brazelton Neonatal Behavior Assessment Scale (BNBAS; completed by professional)	▶ Assesses social and interactive behavior of newborns from birth to 1 month ▶ May be used to examine early individual differences in infants ▶ Has been used in nursing as a strategy for teaching parents about newborn capabilities	Examination guide contains 27 reflex items, 27 behavioral response items, and ratings of infant's predominant states, need for stimulation, and self-quieting activities. Typical exam requires 30 minutes. Training is necessary to establish skill in evaluation.
Neonatal Perception Inventories (NPI; parent self-report)	▶ Measures maternal perception of newborn, comparing a hypothetical "average" baby with perception of own baby. Based on the assumption that a mother ideally will rate her own newborn better than average.	Written scale asks for rating of own baby and average baby on six characteristics; sleeping, feeding, spitting up, elimination, crying, and predictability of behavior. Useful in combination with other assessments of maternal-newborn relationships.
Home Observation Measurement of Environment (HOME, birth to 3 years; completed by professional)	▶ Identifies aspects of environmental that enhance development of infants	Comprises observation of 1 hour in home on six subscales focusing on maternal responsiveness and organization of physical (especially play) environment.

(*Source:* May, K. A., & Maklmeister, L. R. [1990]. *Comprehensive maternity nursing: Nursing process and the childbearing family* [2nd ed.] Philadelphia: J. B. Lippincott.)

1. North American Nursing Diagnosis Association (NANDA) nursing diagnosis categories that could apply to the mother, father, or family include:
   a. Anxiety
   b. Constipation
   c. Ineffective Breast-feeding
   d. Family Coping: High Risk for Growth
   e. Ineffective Family Coping: Compromised
   f. Decisional Conflict
   g. Fatigue
   h. Fear
   i. Anticipatory Grieving
   j. Dysfunctional Grieving
   k. Altered Health Maintenance
   l. High Risk for Infection
   m. Knowledge Deficit
   n. Altered Nutrition: Less than Body Requirements, More than Body Requirements
   o. Pain
   p. Altered Parenting
   q. Self-concept Disturbance
   r. Altered Patterns of Sexuality
   s. Altered Patterns of Urinary Elimination
2. Nursing diagnoses applicable to the neonate could include:
   a. High Risk for Altered Body Temperature
   b. Ineffective Breathing Pattern
   c. Diarrhea
   d. High Risk for Infection
   e. Altered Nutrition: Less than Body Requirements, More than Body Requirements
   f. Pain
   g. Impaired Tissue Integrity
3. Pertinent collaborative problems could include:
   a. Potential Complication: Sepsis
   b. Potential Complication (of circumcision): Hemorrhage, Hypothermia.

C. Planning and implementation
1. Nursing intervention in maternal-newborn care involves activities designed to move the patient or family toward increased positive adaptation and high-level wellness, encompassing everything from administering comfort measures to counseling and health education.
2. Dissemination of the plan for care to others responsible for providing care is essential to providing continuity and safety.
3. Specific patient problems, interventions, and expected outcomes for each problem need to be documented.

8

4. Patient teaching for self-care is a primary nursing intervention with healthy childbearing families.
5. Patient teaching for self-care is based on such considerations as:
    a. Patient or family learning needs
    b. Principles of teaching and learning
    c. Physical and psychological condition of patient and family
    d. Sociocultural factors

D. Evaluation
1. Appropriate evaluation involves:
    a. Establishing criteria to observe and measure
    b. Assessing the present response for evidence
    c. Comparing the present response to the established criteria
2. Any statement of the effectiveness and reliability of nursing actions is best made with qualifications indicating the degree or amount of effectiveness and the reliability claimed.
3. Nursing evaluation of actual outcomes may then result in a reassessment and adjustment in the plan of care or in a refocusing on other identified problems.

Bibliography

May, K. A., & Mahlmeister, L. R. (1990). *Comprehensive maternity nursing: Nursing process and the childbearing family* (2nd ed.). Philadelphia: J. B. Lippincott.

Reeder, S. J., & Martin, L. L. (1987). *Maternity nursing: Family, newborn, and women's health care* (16th ed.). Philadelphia: J. B. Lippincott.

STUDY QUESTIONS

1. The 1935 Amendment to Title V of the Social Security Act accomplished which of the following?
   a. established nurse–midwifery in the United States
   b. marked the first federal involvement in maternity care
   c. emphasized comprehensive prenatal and infant care in public clinics
   d. provided federal funding for maternal-child health in response to priorities set by a national commission

2. All of the following would be considered features of comprehensive family-centered birth care *except*
   a. transfer from labor room to delivery room for birth
   b. prenatal and parent education opportunities
   c. accommodation for presence of support person at a complicated or cesarean birth
   d. early postbirth discharge and planned follow-up care

3. According to the National Commission of Nursing Implementation Project: A Projection of the Immediate Future in Health Care (1986), all of the following are forces that are seen as impacting the health care delivery system of the future *except*
   a. increasing quality of college applicants
   b. shifting payment systems
   c. government interventions in cost containment
   d. technology explosion

4. For many centuries, childbirth typically occurred in the home. In which of the following centuries did a majority of babies begin to be born in hospital settings?
   a. 17th century
   b. 18th century
   c. 19th century
   d. 20th century

5. An important program initiated in the mid-1970s, which provides supplemental foods and nutrition education to low-income families, is represented by which of the following acronyms?
   a. CHAP
   b. EPSDT
   c. WIC
   d. CNM

6. Which of the following is more typical of traditional care in maternity nursing?
   a. homelike atmosphere for birth
   b. early parent–infant contact
   c. scheduling of infant feedings and routines
   d. father participation as coach

7. Increased litigation has occurred in maternal-child care in the past 15 years. The most commonly filed lawsuit involves which of the following claims?
   a. birth injury to the infant related to substandard care
   b. maternal injury as a result of cesarean section delivery
   c. maternal death resulting from physician error
   d. infant death related to physician and nurse incompetence

8. Which agency was founded and authorized by Congress in 1962 to support research and training in basic research relating to prenatal development?
   a. The National Center for Family Planning
   b. The National Institute of Child Health and Human Development
   c. The Department of Health, Education, and Welfare
   d. The Department of Health and Human Services

9. The Frontier Nursing Service provided the first organized midwifery service in the United States. It was founded in 1925 by
   a. Lillian D. Wald
   b. Lavinia L. Dock
   c. Isabel Hampton Robb
   d. Mary Breckinridge

10. Nonviolent or gentle birth practices are primarily associated with
    a. Leboyer
    b. Lemaze
    c. Bowlby
    d. Dick-Reed

ANSWER KEY

1. **Correct response: d**
   The 1935 Amendment to Title V provided federal funding for maternal-child health care.
   a. Organized nurse–midwifery grew out of the activities of the Maternity Association in New York City.
   b. The Sheppard-Towner Act of 1921 marked the first federal involvement in maternity care.
   c. The The Maternal and Infant Care (MIC) projects emphasized comprehensive prenatal and infant care in public clinics.
   Knowledge/Health promotion/NA

2. **Correct response: a**
   Transfer from labor room to delivery room is a characteristic of traditional care.
   b, c, and d. These are all characteristics of family-centered maternity care.
   Knowledge/Health promotion/NA

3. **Correct response: a**
   It is, in fact, the *declining* pool of college applicants that is cited as a factor impacting on future health care delivery.
   b, c, and d. These are all current trends in health care.
   Knowledge/Health promotion/NA

4. **Correct response: d**
   It was not until the 1900s that the majority of births occurred in hospitals.
   a, b, and c. These time frames are all too early.
   Knowledge/Health promotion/NA

5. **Correct response: c**
   The WIC (Women, Infants, and Children) program deals with food and nutrition.
   a. CHAP refers to the Child Health Assessment Act.
   b. EPSDT is the Early and Periodic Screening Diagnostic and Treatment program.
   d. CNM stands for certified nurse–midwife.
   Comprehensive/Health promotion/NA

6. **Correct response: c**
   Rigid scheduling of infant feeding and care routines is an example of traditional maternity nursing.
   a, b, and d. These aspects are more typical of family-centered birth care.
   Comprehensive/Health promotion/Planning

7. **Correct response: a**
   Birth injury with long-term consequences is most frequently claimed in obstetrical law suits.
   b, c, and d. These claims are all less common than birth injury.
   Comprehensive/Safe care/NA

8. **Correct response: b**
   The National Institute of Child Health and Human Development was established in 1962 to support research involving prenatal development.
   a. The NCFP was established in 1969 under HEW to serve as a clearing house for contraceptive information.
   c. HEW was established in 1953, encompassing major programs in public health, education, and economic security.
   d. HHS was established in 1980 to protect and advance the health of the American people.
   Knowledge/NA/NA

9. **Correct response: d**
   Mary Breckinridge founded the Frontier Nursing Service in 1925.
   a. Lillian Wald established, among other things, the House on Henry Street and initiated public school nursing in 1902.
   b. Lavinia Dock was a prominent suffragist and feminist.
   c. Isabel Hamptom Robb organized the Johns Hopkins Hospital school of nursing and was a founder of the American Journal of Nursing.
   Knowledge/NA/NA

10. *Correct response: a*

Dr. Frederick Leboyer, a French obstetrician, suggested new delivery room procedures to make birth a less traumatic event for the newborn.

b. Lamaze is generally associated with natural childbirth practices.

c. John Bowlby described the impact of maternal deprivation on children.

d. Grantly Dick-Reed introduced the concept of prepared childbirth.

Knowledge/NA/NA

Sexuality and Reproduction

I. Overview
A. Sexuality
1. A person's sexuality encompasses the complex of emotions, attitudes, preferences, and behaviors related to expression of the sexual self and eroticism.
2. Sex is a dynamic aspect of life, intertwined with biologic and psychosocial components that cannot be separated.
3. Nurses commonly serve as resource persons for patients seeking information relating to human sexuality and functioning during the reproductive years.

4. Developmental tasks of sexual identity include:
    a. Gender identity: sense of masculinity and femininity; established in part by how the patient was treated by his or her parents as a child
    b. Sex role standards: behavior, attributes, and attitudes that differentiate roles
    c. Sexual partner preference: may be heterosexual, homosexual, or bisexual; may vary during lifetime; probably shaped by complex interaction of several factors, including prenatal hormone environment, early parent interactions, social mores and values, family dynamics, and imitation of most valued parent
5. Responsible sexuality involves commitment to a relationship, responsible reproductive health care, and rational decisions about childbearing.

B. Male and female reproductive potentials
   1. A woman's reproductive lifespan is finite; it begins shortly after menarche, declines somewhat during the late reproductive years, and terminates with menopause—typically a span of 35 to 40 years.
   2. The large initial store of germ cells (primordial ova) present at birth represent the total ova formed during the lifespan. By way of the process of atresia, these germ cells decrease in number; by puberty, only 300,000 of the 6 to 7 million fetal germ cells remain. A woman releases no more than 500 ova during ovulation throughout her lifetime.
   3. A woman's capacity to reproduce may be disassociated from sexual excitement or receptivity.
   4. Reproductive activity in the male begins with sperm production at the onset of puberty and continues throughout his lifespan.
   5. New sperm cells are generated every 74 days, and billions of mature sperm are produced during a man's normal lifespan.
   6. A man's capacity to reproduce is associated with sexual excitement, penile erection, and ejaculation.

II. Female reproductive system
   A. External organs
   1. Mons pubis: a mound of fatty tissue over the symphysis pubis that cushions and protects the bone
   2. Labia majora: longitudinal folds of pigmented skin extending from the mons pubis to the perineum
   3. Labia minora: soft longitudinal skin folds between the labia majora
   4. Clitoris: erectile tissue located at upper end of labia minora; primary site of sexual arousal
   5. Urethral meatus (urethral orifice): small opening of urethra lo-

cated between clitoris and vaginal orifice for the purpose of urination

6. Skene's or paraurethral glands: small mucous glands that open into posterior wall of the urinary meatus and provide vaginal lubrication
7. Vestibule: an almond-shaped area between the labia minora containing the vaginal introitus, hymen, and Bartholin's glands
8. Vaginal introitus: external opening of the vagina
9. Hymen: membranous tissue ringing the vaginal introitus
10. Bartholin's or vulvovaginal glands: mucus-secreting glands located on either side of the vaginal orifice
11. Perineal body: muscles and fascia that support pelvic structures
12. Perineum: tissue between the anus and vagina; the area where episiotomy is performed

B. Internal organs

1. Vagina: the female organ of copulation, a tubular musculomembranous organ lying between the rectum and the urethra and bladder; also known as the birth canal
2. Uterus: a hollow muscular organ with three muscle layers (perimetrium, myometrium, and endometrium) located between the bladder and rectum and consisting of three parts: fundus, body (corpus), and cervix; uterine functions include:
    a. Menstruation: sloughing away of spongy layers of endometrium with bleeding from torn vessels
    b. Pregnancy: development of embryo and fetus after fertilization
    c. Labor: powerful contractions of muscular uterine wall that result in expulsion of fetus
3. Uterine ligaments include:
    a. Broad and round ligaments, which provide upper support for the uterus
    b. Cardinal, pubocervical, and uterosacral ligaments, which are suspensory and provide middle support
    c. Pelvic muscular floor ligaments, which provide lower support
4. Fallopian tubes: tubes extending from the upper outer angles of the uterus and end near the ovary; serve as passageway for the ovum from the ovary to the uterus and for the sperm from the uterus to the ovary
5. Ovaries: female sex glands located on each side of the uterus with two functions:
    a. Ovulation (release of ovum)
    b. Secretion of hormones (estrogen and progesterone)

C. Pelvis

1. The pelvis is a bony ring located in lower portion of the trunk,

consisting of three parts (ilium, ischium, and pubis) and four bones (two innominate bones, or hipbones, sacrum, and coccyx).

2. The pelvic bones are held together by four joints (articulations): symphysis pubis, two sacroiliac, and sacrococcygeal; fibrocartilage between these joints provides for movability.

3. Type of pelves include:
   a. Gynecoid: typical female pelvis with rounded inlet
   b. Android: normal male pelvis with heart-shaped inlet
   c. Anthropoid: "ape-like" pelvis with oval inlet
   d. Platypelloid: flat female-type pelvis with transverse oval inlet

4. Pelvic structural irregularities can alter labor.

5. Pelvimetry (internal or external measurements), obtained by a pelvimeter, radiography, or internal examination, include:
   a. Internal pelvic inlet measurement: diagonal conjugate—lower margin of symphysis pubis to promontory of sacrum—normally 12.5 to 13 cm
   b. Internal midpelvic measurement: distance between ischial spines and prominence or bluntness of spines, normally 10.5 cm
   c. Internal pelvic outlet measurement: estimation of width of pubic arch, mobility of coccyx, intertuberous diameter, and posterior sagittal diameter

D. Breasts

1. The female breasts (mammary glands) are specialized sebaceous glands that produce milk after childbirth (lactation).

2. Internal breast structures include:
   a. Glandular tissue (parenchyma): acini (milk-producing cells), which cluster in groups of 15 to 20 to form the lobes of the breast
   b. Lactiferous ducts or sinuses, which form passageways from the lobes to the nipple
   c. Fibrous tissue: Cooper's ligaments, which provide support to the mammary glands
   d. Adipose and fibrous tissue (stroma), which provide the relative size and consistency of the breast

3. External structures include:
   a. Nipple: raised, pigmented area of the breast
   b. Areola: pigmented skin around nipple
   c. Montgomery's tubercles: sebaceous glands of the areola

4. The breasts change in size and nodularity in response to ovarian cycle hormonal changes, including:
   a. Estrogen stimulation, producing tenderness
   b. Progesterone (postovulation), causing increased tenderness and breast enlargement

5. Physical changes in breast size and activity are at a minimum 5 to 7 days after menstruation stops; this is the best time to detect pathologic changes through breast self-examination.

E. Menstrual cycle

1. The menstrual cycle is a monthly cyclical pattern of ovulation and menstruation involving:
   a. Ovulation: discharge of mature ovum from ovary
   b. Menstruation: periodic shedding of blood and mucous epithelial cells from uterus
2. Menarche (onset of menstruation) typically occurs between age 12 and 14 years.
3. The ovary produces mature gametes and secretes the following hormones:
   a. Estrogen: contributes to characteristics of femaleness (e.g., female body build, breast growth)
   b. Progesterone (hormone of pregnancy): quiets or decreases contractility of the uterus
   c. Prostaglandins: regulate reproductive process (stimulate contractility of uterine and other smooth muscles)
4. The menstrual cycle occurs in four levels: CNS level (hypothalamic–pituitary), ovarian level, endometrial (menstrual) level, and the cervical level.
5. At the CNS level:
   a. The hypothalamus stimulates the anterior pituitary by secreting gonadotropin-releasing hormone (GnRH); the anterior pituitary secretes two gonadotropins—follicle-stimulating hormone (FSH) and luteinizing hormone (LH).
   b. FSH stimulates the ovary to develop ovarian follicles; the developing follicles secrete estrogen, which feeds back to the anterior pituitary to suppress FSH and trigger an LH surge.
   c. LH acts with FSH to cause ovulation and enhance corpus luteum formation.
6. At the ovarian level:
   a. An oocyte grows within the primordial follicle in two phases: follicular phase and luteal phase.
   b. In the follicular phase (days 1 to 14), the follicle matures due to FSH.
   c. In the luteal phase (days 15 to 22), the corpus luteum develops from a ruptured follicle.
7. The endometrial level involves:
   a. Menstrual phase (days 1 to 5), during which the estrogen level is low and cervical mucus is scanty
   b. Proliferative (follicular) phase (days 6 to 14), during which the estrogen level is high, the endometrium and myome-

trium thicken, and changes in cervical mucosa occur (note: variations in the menstrual cycle are due to variations in the number of days in this phase)

    c.   Secretory phase (days 14 to 26): following release of ovum, estrogen level drops, progesterone level is high, increased uterine vascularity occurs, and tissue glycogen levels increase

    d.   Ischemic phase (days 27 to 28), involving low estrogen and progesterone levels, arterial vasoconstriction, pallor of endometrium, and blood vessel rupture

  8.   The cervical level involves:

    a.   Preovulation: increased estrogen level causes cervical os dilatation, abundant liquid mucus, high spinnbarkheit, excellent sperm penetration

    b.   Postovulation: increased progesterone level results in cervical os constriction, scant viscous mucus, low spinnbarkheit, no ferning, poor sperm penetration

    c.   During pregnancy: increased circulation

G. **Climacteric**

  1.   The climacteric is a transitional period during which ovarian function and hormonal production decline.

  2.   Menopause refers to a woman's last menstrual period; the average age of menopause is 52 years.

  3.   Women may ovulate after menopause and thus can become pregnant.

III. **Male reproductive system**

  A. **External structures**

    1.   Penis: the male organ of copulation; a cylindrical shaft consisting of:

      a.   Two lateral columns of erectile tissue (corpora cavernosa)

      b.   A column of erectile tissue on the underside of the penis (corpus spongiosum) that encases the urethra

      c.   The glans penis, a cone-shaped expansion of the corpus spongiosum that is highly sensitive to sexual stimulus

      d.   The prepuce, or foreskin, a skin flap that covers the glans penis in uncircumcised males

    2.   Scrotum: a pouch hanging below the penis that contains the testes. Internally, the medial septum divides the scrotum into two sacs, each of which contains a testis.

  B. **Internal structures**

    1.   Testis: two solid ovoid organs 4 to 5 cm long, divided into lobes containing seminiferous tubules, where spermatogenesis occurs; functions include production of testosterone and spermatogenesis

    2.   Epididymis: a tubular sac located next to each testis that serves as reservoir for sperm storage and maturation

3. Vas deferens: a duct extending from the epididymis to the ejaculatory duct, providing a passageway for sperm
4. Ejaculatory duct: the canal formed by the union of the vas deferens and the excretory duct of the seminal vesicle, which enters the urethra at the prostate gland
5. Urethra: the passageway for both urine and semen, extending from the bladder to the urethral meatus

C. **Accessory glands**
1. Other structures in the male reproductive system produce secretions that facilitate transportation of spermatozoa along the urethra during ejaculation and also provide a temporary safe milieu for the fragile sperm. The function of the accessory glands is maintained by testosterone.
2. Seminal vesicles: located behind the bladder and in front of the rectum, deliver secretions to the urethra through the ejaculatory ducts
3. Prostate gland: surrounds the base of the urethra and the ejaculatory duct; secretes a clear fluid with a slightly acid pH rich in acid phosphatase, citric acid, zinc, and proteolytic enzymes
4. Bulbourethral and urethral glands (Cowper's glands): lie at the base of the prostate and on either side of the membranous urethra, and produce a clear, alkaline mucinous substance that lubricates the urethra and coats its surface; the alkalinity assists in neutralizing the acidic female vaginal secretions, which would be detrimental to sperm survival

D. **Semen**
1. Semen is a thick, whitish fluid ejaculated by the male during orgasm; contains spermatozoa and fructose-rich nutrients.
2. During ejaculation, semen receives contributions of fluid from the seminal vesicles and the prostate gland.
3. Combined semen is alkaline (average pH, 7.5).
4. The average amount of semen released during ejaculation is 3 to 5 mL.

E. **Male breasts**
1. Male mammary tissue remains dormant throughout life, but the breasts are a site of sexual arousal and excitation.
2. Although rare (accounting for less than 1% of all breast cancers in the United States), male breast cancer occurs frequently enough to warrant routine inspection of the breasts for dimpling, discharge, or nipple inversion.

F. **Neurohormonal control of the male reproductive system**
1. At puberty, the hypothalamus stimulates the pituitary to produce FSH and LH.
2. FSH stimulates germ cells within the testes to manufacture sperm.

3. LH stimulates the production of testosterone in the testes.
4. Testosterone, one of several androgens (and the most potent) produced in the testes, is responsible for the development of secondary sex characteristics at puberty.
5. Testosterone production occurs in the interstitial cells of Leydig, in the seminiferous tubules. Leydig cells are abundant in the newborn and pubescent male, and testosterone is abundant during these periods. Testosterone production slows after age 40 years; by age 80, production is only about one fifth of peak level.
6. Although LH stimulates the Leydig cells to produce testosterone from cholesterol, testosterone inhibits the secretion of LH by the anterior pituitary.
7. Spermatogenesis (sperm production) occurs continually after puberty, providing large numbers of sperm for unlimited ejaculations over the mature lifespan.
8. Spermatozoa are released from the epithelial wall of the seminiferous tubules. Meiosis occurs during the process, and the number of chromosomes in each cell is reduced by one half (haploid number).
9. Spermatogenesis is a heat-sensitive process; the 2 to 3 degrees of difference between scrotal and abdominal temperatures allows spermatogenesis to proceed in the cooler environment.
10. The entire period of spermatogenesis, from germinal cell to mature sperm, takes about 75 days.

IV. Sexual response
A. Female sexual response cycle
1. During the *excitement phase*:
   a. Vaginal lubrication occurs.
   b. The inner two-thirds of the vagina begin to lengthen and distend, and the outer one-third undergoes slight thickening.
   c. The body of the uterus is pulled upward.
   d. The vaginal walls become congested with blood and darken in color.
   e. The clitoris increases in diameter, possibly with slightly increased tumescence of the glans clitoris.
   f. The labia minora become engorged with blood and increase in size.
   g. The labia majora tend to flatten somewhat and retract away from the middle of the vulva.
   h. The nipples become erect and breast size increases.
   i. Flushing occurs in approximately 75% of females.
   j. Overall muscle tension increases.
2. In the *plateau phase*:
   a. The walls of the outer one-third of the vagina become fur-

ther engorged with blood, decreasing the internal vaginal diameter.
b. The labia minora become further engorged with blood and darken and swell.
c. The clitoris retracts and is covered by the clitoral hood; the clitoral body decreases in size by about 50%.
d. The nipples become further engorged.
e. Flushing may spread to the abdomen, thighs, and back.
f. A further increase in muscle tension occurs; breathing becomes deeper; heart rate and blood pressure increase markedly as tension rises toward orgasm.

3. The *orgasmic phase* is marked by:
a. Strong muscular contractions in the outer one third of the vagina, with the inner two thirds tending to expand
b. Contraction of uterine muscles
c. No observable changes in labia majora, labia minora, clitoris, or breasts
d. Flushing reaching a peak of color intensity and distribution
e. Possibly strong muscular contractions, both voluntary and involuntary, in many parts of the body, including rectal sphincter muscle
f. Respiratory rate possibly reaching a peak of two to three times normal, heart rate possibly doubling, and blood pressure increasing as much as one-third above normal

4. During *resolution*:
a. Blood engorging the walls of the outer one third of the vagina disperses rapidly.
b. The inner two thirds of the vagina gradually shrink, and color returns to preexcitement shade.
c. The uterus descends toward the vaginal barrel.
d. The labia minora and majora return to unstimulated thickness and close toward midline.
e. The clitoris protrudes from under the clitoral hood, and eventually returns to prestimulated size.
f. Flushing disappears.
g. Muscles relax quickly.
h. Heart rate and blood pressure return to normal.

B. Male sexual response cycle
1. In the *excitement phase*:
a. Penile erection begins.
b. Scrotal skin becomes congested and thick.
c. Testes elevate into the scrotal sac.
d. Some nipple erection may occur.
e. Flushing may occur.
f. Heart rate and blood pressure begin to increase.

       g.   Generalized increase in muscle tension occurs, with a tendency toward involuntary muscle contractions.

2.   The *plateau phase* is marked by:
- a.   Further increase in size of penis, sometimes with color changes corresponding to reddening of female labia
- b.   Possible preorgasmic emission, thought to come from Cowper's glands
- c.   Continued testicular elevation, increase in size of testes, and rotation of testes (approximately 30 degrees)
- d.   Further increase in heart rate and blood pressure; increased respiratory rate
- e.   Increased muscle tension

3.   During the *orgasmic phase*:
- a.   Rhythmic contractions expel semen from the epididymis through the vas deferens, seminal vesicles, prostate gland, urethra, and out the urethral meatus.
- b.   Testes are at maximum elevation, size, and rotation.
- c.   Flushing reaches its peak.
- d.   Heart and respiratory rates also peak.
- e.   A general loss of voluntary control occurs.
- f.   A refractory period begins as the final contractions of the urethral walls occur.

4.   In the *resolution phase*:
- a.   More than 50% of the erection is lost rapidly in the first stage of resolution, with the penis gradually returning to its unstimulated size during the second stage.
- b.   The scrotum gradually loses its congested and thick status.
- c.   The testes descend and return to normal size.
- d.   Nipple erection subsides.
- e.   Flushing disappears.
- f.   Heart rate, blood pressure, and respiratory rate return to normal.
- g.   General muscle relaxation occurs.

C.   Differences in male and female sexual response

1.   Women have three identifiable sexual response patterns:
- a.   Rapid progression to plateau stage with some peaks and valleys, and one intense orgasm followed by rapid resolution; resembles the male pattern
- b.   Steady progression to plateau stage followed by an intense orgasm and possibly subsequent orgasms, with slower resolution
- c.   Slower progression to plateau stage followed by minor surges toward orgasm, causing prolonged pleasurable feelings without definitive orgasm

2.   Males have one basic sexual response pattern: excitement pro-

gresses steadily to plateau stage, with one intense orgasm followed by resolution.

3. In general, women experience orgasms in a wider range of duration and intensity than do men.

4. Female orgasmic contractions last twice as long as the male's; the strength of the contractions is not as markedly concentrated in the first few pulsations.

D. Sexual concerns related to pregnancy

1. During pregnancy, the woman's desire for sex may be altered due to fatigue, nausea, and other discomforts of pregnancy.

2. Other common sexual concerns during pregnancy include dyspareunia and male erectile dysfunction.

3. Breasts may be painful to touch, especially during the first trimester.

4. Some men may find the normal increase in the amount and odor of vaginal discharge during pregnancy a "turn off"; others, however, do not share this distaste.

5. Some women and couples need "permission" to be sexually active during pregnancy, along with reassurance that female orgasm will not harm the fetus.

6. For a couple who cannot have or who choose not to have intercourse during pregnancy, kissing, hugging, and oral or manual genital stimulation can be satisfying expressions of closeness and intimacy.

V. Implications for nursing

A. Assessment

1. Before interacting with any patient regarding sexuality and reproduction, the nurse must perform a self-assessment; personal attitudes and values will greatly influence the nursing care provided.

2. A sexual history involves gathering information about the patient's or couple's:
   a. Past and current experiences with sex
   b. Sexual knowledge and how it was obtained
   c. Attitudes toward sexuality
   d. Current problem, if any

B. Nursing diagnoses

1. Anxiety
2. Body Image Disturbance
3. Ineffective Individual Coping
4. Knowledge Deficit
5. Self-esteem Disturbance
6. Sexual Dysfunction
7. Altered Sexuality Patterns

C. Planning and implementation

1. Create a private, trusting milieu to encourage patients to discuss sexual issues openly.

24

    2.   Validate and reassure patients about the universality of their sexual concerns.

    3.   Provide information about alternate means of sexual expression, as appropriate.

    4.   Refer patients with complex problems to professionals specializing in sexuality issues.

D. Evaluation

    1.   The patient or couple verbalizes mutual satisfaction with choices regarding sexuality.

    2.   The patient or couple continues to make adjustments regarding sexuality throughout the pregnancy.

Bibliography

May, K. A., & Mahlmeister, L. R. (1990). *Comprehensive maternity nursing: Nursing process and the childbearing family* (2nd ed.). Philadelphia: J. B. Lippincott.

Reeder, S. J., & Martin, L. L. (1987). *Maternity nursing: Family, newborn, and women's health care* (16th ed.). Philadelphia: J. B. Lippincott.

STUDY QUESTIONS

1. Days 6 through 14 of the menstrual cycle, under the influence of estrogen secreted by the ovary, are known as which of the following phases?
   a. estrogen
   b. follicular
   c. luteal
   d. proliferative

2. Three layers of involuntary muscles—longitudinal, interlacing, and circular—comprise which uterine layer?
   a. decidua
   b. endometrium
   c. myometrium
   d. perimetrium

3. The region between the vaginal orifice and the anus is known as the
   a. mons
   b. perineum
   c. peritoneum
   d. vestibule

4. Which breast structure is responsible for milk production?
   a. acini
   b. areola
   c. lactiferous ducts
   d. Montgomery's tubercles

5. Gonadotropic hormones are released by the pituitary gland under the regulation of the
   a. adrenal
   b. hypothalamus
   c. thalamus
   d. thyroid

6. Which pituitary hormone stimulates the ovary to produce estrogen during the menstrual cycle?
   a. follicle-stimulating hormone (FSH)
   b. gonadotropin-releasing hormone (GnRH)
   c. luteinizing hormone (LH)
   d. human chorionic gonadotropin (HCG)

7. During the menstrual cycle, ovulation generally occurs
   a. 7 days after the last day of the menstrual period
   b. 14 days after the last day of the menstrual cycle
   c. 7 days before the end of menstruation
   d. 14 days before the end of the menstrual cycle

8. Variations in the length of the menstrual cycle are due to the variations in the number of days in the
   a. follicular phase
   b. luteal phase
   c. ischemic phase
   d. secretory phase

9. A patient asks the nurse "What is the normal amount of blood loss during menstruation?" What would be the nurse's best response?
   a. "Normal blood loss can vary from a little to a lot."
   b. "Normal blood loss is about 120 mL."
   c. "Normal blood loss is about ¼ cup."
   d. "Normal blood loss is about ⅛ cup."

ANSWER KEY

26

1. *Correct response: b*
    During the follicular phase, the ovarian follicle is growing.
    a. Estrogen is not a phase of the menstrual cycle, but rather a hormone produced by the ovary.
    c. During the luteal phase, the corpus luteum develops.
    d. During this phase of the menstrual cycle, endometrial glands enlarge in response to estrogen.
    Comprehensive/Safe care/Assessment

2. *Correct response: c*
    The myometrium is the uterine muscular layer.
    a. The decidua is the mucous lining of the uterus during pregnancy.
    b. The endometrium is the inner mucous membrane of the uterus.
    d. The perimetrium is the outer layer of the uterine corpus.
    Comprehensive/Physiologic/Assessment

3. *Correct response: b*
    The perineum is the region between the vaginal orifice and anus.
    a. The mons is fatty tissue over the symphysis pubis.
    c. The peritoneum is the membrane over the viscera and lining the abdominal cavity.
    d. The vestibule is the area between the labia minora.
    Knowledge/Physiologic/Assessment

4. *Correct response: a*
    Acini are cells in the breast are responsible for milk production.
    b. The areola is to the pigmented area around the nipple.
    c. Lactiferous ducts transport milk to the nipple for feeding.
    d. Montgomery's tubercles are small nodules around the nipple on the areola.
    Knowledge/Safe care/Assessment

5. *Correct response: b*
    The hypothalamus controls pituitary release of gonadotropic hormones.
    a. The adrenal gland, located on the surface of the kidney, produces adrenocorticoid hormones.
    c. This gland, located in the wall of the third ventricle, receives sensory impulses.
    d. The thyroid is a gland of internal secretion in the neck.
    Knowledge/Safe care/Assessment

6. *Correct response: a*
    FSH is a pituitary hormone that stimulates the ovary.
    b. GnRH is a hormone released by the hypothalamus.
    c. LH is a hormone released by chorionic villi.
    d. HCG is a gonad-stimulating hormone secreted by the placenta during fetal development.
    Knowledge/Safe care/Assessment

7. *Correct response: d*
    The most stable period of the menstrual cycle extends from 14 days from ovulation to the beginning of menstruation due to the stability of the luteal phase.
    a, b, and c. These responses are incorrect.
    Knowledge/Safe care/Assessment

8. *Correct response: a*
    Variation in the follicular phase affects the length of the menstrual cycle.
    b. This is the stable ovarian phase.
    c and d. These are part of the uterine phase.
    Comprehensive/Safe care/Assessment

9. *Correct response: c*
    Normal blood loss during menstruation is about 30 mL, or ¼ cup (explained in a common measure).
    a. This response is too vague and provides no useful information to the patient.
    b. One cup or 120 mL of blood loss is excessive.
    d. Only ⅛ cup or 15 mL of blood loss is too scant, and could stimulate ovulation.
    Application/Physiologic/Implementation

Fetal Growth and Development

I. Conception

A. Fertilization

1. Fertilization refers to impregnation by union of an ovum and a spermatozoan.

2. Following ejaculation into the vagina, sperm live approximately 48 hours; after ovulation, the ovum remains fertile for 10 to 15 hours. Thus, for fertilization to occur, coitus must be accomplished no more than 48 hours before before or 15 hours after ovulation.

3. Fertilization occurs in the ampulla (outer one third) of the fallopian tube following ovulation.

4. Increased estrogen levels at the time of ovulation provide three functions:
   a. Increase the fallopian tube's ability to contract and move the ovum down the tube
   b. Cause thinning of cervical mucus, facilitating sperm penetration
   c. Stimulate growth of uterine muscle (myometrium) and glandular epithelium (endometrium), and induce the synthesis of receptors for progesterone
5. Progesterone acts on the estrogen-primed endometrium to convert it to actively secreting tissue; progesterone also:
   a. Causes the cervical mucus to become thick and sticky (i.e., the mucus plug), which protects the fetus against invading bacteria
   b. Decreases motility of oviducts and uterus
   c. Stimulates glandular breast tissue growth
6. Complex changes in hormone blood levels provide the basis for diagnostic tests of fetal maturity and well-being.
7. The corpus luteum provides most of the estrogen and progesterone during the first 2 months of gestation. Persistence of the corpus luteum and these two steroid hormones is essential to sustain the uterine endometrium and prevent menstruation.
8. Chorionic gonadotropin (CG), a hormone secreted by the blastocyst and placenta, is partly responsible for the maintenance of the corpus luteum. Detection of CG in the urine or plasma provides the basis of most pregnancy tests.
9. Estriol, a major estrogen of pregnancy, depends on the presence of a fetal adrenal enzyme for its synthesis; thus, measurement of maternal estriol levels provides a means of monitoring fetal well-being.

B. Multiple pregnancy
1. Approximately 2% of births in the United States are multiple. Most involve twins; triplets occur in one of 7600 pregnancies. Multiple births higher than triplets are rare, but the incidence is rising due to the increasing use of gonadotropins to treat women with ovulatory failure.
3. Dizygotic (fraternal) multiple pregnancy involves two or more ova fertilized by separate sperm. Fetuses have separate placentas, amnions, and chorions (although the placenta may fuse together to resemble a single one), and may be the same or different sexes.
4. Monozygotic (identical) multiple pregnancy develops from a single fertilized ovum. Fetuses share a common placenta and chorion, but have separate amnions; they are the same sex and have the same genotype.

II. Stages of growth and development
A. Essential concepts
1. Factors influencing embryonic and fetal development include:
   a. Environmental (e.g., poverty, maternal drug or alcohol use, malnutrition)
   b. Anatomic problems:
      (1) Maternal (e.g., ectopic pregnancy, uterine abnormality, retroversion of uterus, incompetent cervical os)
      (2) Fetal (e.g., chromosomal defect, poor implantation)
   c. Maternal complications (e.g., infection, Rh incompatibility, cyanotic heart disease, renal diseases, hypertension, urinary tract infection)
   d. Fetal complications (e.g., premature rupture of membranes, preterm labor, postmaturity)
   e. Physiologic (e.g., folate deficiency, endocrine deficiency, defective sperm)
2. Fetal development occurs in three stages: pre-embryonic, embryonic, and fetal. (Table 3–1 shows a breakdown of fetal development by gestational month.)

B. Pre-embryonic stage
1. Encompassing the first 14 days after conception, this stage is characterized by rapid growth and differentiation, and establishment of embryonic membranes and germ layers.
2. Implantation of blastocyst occurs approximately 7 to 9 days after fertilization.
3. Endometrium becomes the decidua following conception and implantation.
4. Two embryonic membranes form to protect and support the embryo:
   a. Chorion, the outside embryonic membrane
   b. Amnion, the innermost membrane
5. All tissues and organs develop from the three primary germ layers of the embryo:
   a. Ectoderm: central nervous system; peripheral nervous system; sensory epithelium of ear, nose, eye, sinus, mouth, and anal canal; skin (epidermis), hair, nails, sebaceous glands, sweat glands, hair follicles; mammary glands, pituitary gland, enamel of teeth and oral glands
   b. Mesoderm: bone, cartilage, skeleton; connective tissue, smooth and striated muscles; cardiovascular and lymphatic systems; blood and lymph cells; kidneys and reproductive organs; subcutaneous tissues of the skin; serous membrane lining of the pericardial, pleural, and peritoneal cavities; spleen

TABLE 3–1.
Timetable of fetal development

GESTATIONAL MONTH	DEVELOPMENT MILESTONE
1	Fetal length: 0.75 to 1 cm
	Foundations of nervous system, genitourinary system, skin, bones, and lungs form
	Buds of arms and legs start to form
	Rudiments of eyes, ears, and nose appear
2	Fetal length: 2.5 cm; fetal weight: 4 g
	Head is disproportionately large due to brain development
	Sex differentiation begins
	Bone ossification begins
3	Fetal length: 7 to 9 cm; fetal weight: 28 g
	Fingers and toes are formed
	Placental and fetal circulation are complete
4	Fetal length: 10 to 17 cm; fetal weight: 55 to 120 g
	Sex differentiation is completed
	Rudimentary kidneys being to secrete urine
	Heartbeat can be detected
	Nasal septum and palate close
5	Fetal length: 25 cm; fetal weight: 223 g
	Lanugo covers the entire body
	Quickening occurs
	Heart sounds can be ausculated
6	Fetal length: 28 to 36 cm; fetal weight: 680 g
	Vernix caseosa appears
	Eyebrows and fingernails develop
7	Fetal length: 35 to 38 cm; fetal weight: 1200 g
	Pupillary membrane disappears from eyes
	The likelihood of fetal survival in extrauterine environment is good
8	Fetal length: 38 to 43 cm; fetal weight: 2700g
	The fetus is viable
	Eyelids are open
	Vigorous fetal movement occurs
9	Fetal length: 42 to 49 cm; fetal weight: 1900 to 2700 g
	Skin is wrinckled and loose due to subcutaneous fat deposits
	Lanugo disappears
	Amniotic fluid decreases
10	Fetal length: 48 to 52 cm; fetal weight: 3000 g
	Skin is smooth
	Skull bones are ossified and nearly fused at sutures
	Eyes are uniformly slate-colored.

      c.   Endoderm: respiratory tract epithelium, epithelial lining of gastrointestinal tract (pharynx, tongue, tonsils, thyroid, parathyroid, thymus); epithelial lining of urinary bladder and urethra; liver; pancreas

C. **Embryonic stage**
1. This stage begins during the third week after conception and continues until embryo reaches a crown-to-rump length of 3 cm (1.2 in), about the eighth week.
2. This is the period of differentiation of tissues into organs and development of main external features.

D. **Fetal stage**
1. The period from 8 to 10 weeks after conception marks the end of embryonic period and beginning of fetal period.
2. At this time, every structure is present that will be found in the full-term neonate.
3. The remainder of gestational period is devoted to refinement of structures and organization and perfection of function.

E. **Amniotic fluid (bag of waters)**
1. Contained by the amnion membrane that protects the embryo/fetus, this fluid controls temperature, supports symmetrical growth, prevents adherence to amnion, and allows the embryo/fetus to move about the amniotic cavity.
2. Amniotic fluid volume normally ranges from 500 to 1000 mL.

F. **Placenta**
1. The placenta begins to function by the fourth week of gestation; by the 14th week it is a complete, independently functioning organ.
2. It transmits nutrients and oxygen to the fetus and removes waste and carbon dioxide by diffusion.
3. The endocrine organ of pregnancy, the placenta produces:
    a.   Human chorionic gonadotropin (HCG) in maternal blood by day 8 of gestation; produces positive pregnancy test
    b.   Human placental lactogen or human chorionic somatomotropin increases after 20 weeks gestation
    c.   Estrogen: responsible for enhancing growth of all organs by proliferation and nourishment
    d.   Progesterone: responsible for nourishment and relaxation to help maintain pregnancy

III. **Genetic principles**
A. **Chromosome structure**
1. Normal embryonic cell tissue contains 46 chromosomes (23 pairs): 44 homologous (22 pairs) and 2 sex (1 pair) chromosomes.
2. Each chromosome contains 22 autosomes and 1 sex chromosome (Y) from the male and 22 autosomes and 1 sex chromosome (X) from the female.

3. Human life begins as a single cell—zygote—that reproduces itself (as does each new cell).
4. Fetal cells and organs develop from chromosomes; the sex of the embryo is determined from the 1 pair (2 sex chromosomes, one from each parent): female XX and male XY.
5. The sex of the fetus is determined at the time of fertilization by the combination of the sex chromosomes of the sperm (X or Y) and the ovum (Fig. 3–1).
6. By the 12th week of gestation, external genitalia normally are well enough developed to be easily distinguishable.
7. In a female fetus, the fetal ovary has many primordial (primitive) follicles and produces small but increasing amounts of estrogen.
8. The gonads of the genetically male fetus (fetus with Y chromosome) play a critical role information of the genital tract. As the gonads evolve in the testicular pattern—presumably under the influence of maternal HCG and LH and fetal adrenal hormones—the testes produce androgenic hormones that result in growth and differentiation of male genitals.

B.   Chromosomal inheritance
1.   Basic patterns of single-gene inheritance include:
   a.   Autosomal dominant: the clinical expression of a mutant gene in a heterozygous (one allelic gene at a given chromosome locus) individual; disorders include achondroplastic dwarfism
   b.   Autosomal recessive: the clinical expression of a mutant gene when both allelic genes at a given chromosome locus are mutant (homozygous); disorders include cystic fibrosis
   c.   X-linked dominant: rare disorders appearing in every generation of the family. Females, having two X chromosomes, will be symptomatic if heterozygous for an X-linked dominant trait. Males, having only one X chromosome and a Y chromosome, will always be affected if they inherit an X-linked mutant gene.
   d.   X-linked recessive: females will be asymptomatic for trait if

FIGURE 3–1.
Fertilization. (A) Ovum fertilized by X-bearing sperm to form female zygote. (B) Ovum fertilized by Y-bearing sperm to form male zygote.

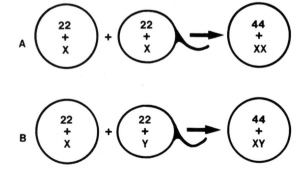

heterozygous for an X-linked recessive trait. Females will manifest symptoms if homozygous for an X-linked recessive disorder. (Note: the terms dominant and recessive in X-linked traits refer only to females.)

2. Multifactorial inheritance involves those traits and disorders resulting from the interaction of many genetic factors (polygenetic inheritance) or the interaction of genetic and environmental factors. Examples of multifactorial disorders include congenital heart defects, clubfoot, neural tube defects, pyloric stenosis, cleft lip and cleft palate, and congenital hip dysplasia.

C. Chromosome disorders (rearrangement)

1. Causes may be hereditary or nonhereditary; contributing factors include internal and environmental events such as exposure to radiation, certain drugs, viruses, toxins and chemicals, and advanced maternal age at conception

2. Types include:
   a. Numerical abnormalities in sex chromosomes and autosomes (e.g., Klinefelter's and Turner's syndromes and Trisomy 13, 18, or 21)
   b. Structural disorders such as deletions (e.g., cri du chat syndrome) and translocations.

IV. Genetic counseling

A. Goals

1. Enable individuals or couples to make informed reproductive decisions.
2. Provide psychological support to assist individuals or couples with decision-making process.
3. Provide clients with information about the defect in question.
4. Communicate to clients the risk of transmitting the defect in question to future conceived children.

B. Screening for genetic traits and disease

1. The goal of screening is to prevent tragic genetic diseases and offer various reproductive options to at-risk couples.
2. Accurate screening hinges on the education and advocacy of physicians and nurses caring for persons of reproductive age, and on accurate identification of the patient's ethnic origin.
3. Specific screens include:
   a. Newborn screening of blood, obtained by heelstick, within 3 to 5 days of birth for presence of phenylketonuria (PKU), maple syrup urine disease, galactosemia, homocystinuria, and tyrosinemia
   b. Maternal serum alpha-fetoprotein (MSAFP) screen, selectively done when an open neural tube defect is suspected (MSAFP is not diagnostic; there is, however, a 5% to 10% risk of the defect when MSAFP is elevated at 16 to 18 weeks' gestation.)

       c.   Heterozygote screening, directed at detecting clinically normal carriers of a disease-causing mutant gene, particularly in persons of ethnic groups known to have a high frequency of the mutant gene under investigation; for example:

           (1)   Tay-Sachs disease in Jews of Eastern European (Ashkenazi) descent

           (2)   Sickle-cell disease in black persons of African descent

           (3)   Beta-thalassemia (Cooley's anemia) in persons of Mediterranean descent (e.g., Italian, Turkish, Sicilian, Sardinian, Greek, Cypriotic)

C.   **Indications for prenatal genetic screening**

    1.   Presence of risk factors for chromosomal disorders, such as:

       a.   Advanced maternal age

       b.   Known carrier parent

       c.   Previous birth of child with chromosomal disorder or with multiple anomalies with no chromosomal studies done

       d.   History of spontaneous abortion

    2.   Known risk for metabolic disorders

    3.   Known risk for sex-linked genetic disorder

    4.   Willingness to consider termination of pregnancy if abnormal fetus is detected

V.   **Implications for nursing (Note: See Chapter 8, Antepartal Care, for information on assessing fetal growth and development.)**

   A.   **Assessment: Obtain a relevant preliminary genetic history, being alert to information indicating the need for referral to genetic counseling.**

   B.   **Nursing diagnoses**

    1.   Decisional Conflict

    2.   Grieving

    3.   Knowledge Deficit

    4.   Self-concept Disturbance

   C.   **Planning and implementation**

    1.   Identify families who need genetic counseling.

    2.   Provide sufficient and correct information about the genetic problem in question.

    3.   Serve as a liaison between the genetic counselor and the family.

    4.   Assist families in coping with the information received; guide them in managing the crisis in their lives.

   D.   **Evaluation**

    1.   Couples of childbearing age from any setting are appropriately screened for genetic problems and given appropriate referral.

    2.   Families faced with difficult decisions with respect to genetic outcomes state that they receive adequate information.

3. Families of childbearing age have access to anticipatory guidance and information.

4. The psychological adaptation of family members to grief and loss related to genetic problems is documented in the nursing process.

Bibliography

Jensen, M. D., & Bobak, I. M. (1985). *Maternity and gynecologic care: The nurse and family* (3rd ed.). St. Louis: C. V. Mosby.

May, K. A., & Mahlmeister, L. R. (1990). *Comprehensive maternity nursing: Nursing process and the childbearing family* (2nd ed.). Philadelphia: J. B. Lippincott.

Olds, S. (1984). *Maternity-newborn nursing*. Menlo Park, CA: Addison-Wesley.

Reeder, S. J., & Martin, L. L. (1987). *Maternity nursing: Family, newborn, and women's health care* (16th ed.). Philadelphia: J. B. Lippincott.

STUDY QUESTIONS

1. The thickened endometrium in which the fertilized embryo implants is called the
   a. endoderm
   b. decidua
   c. amnion
   d. chorion

2. The fetal nervous system is formed by the germ layer known as the
   a. ectoderm
   b. mesoderm
   c. entoderm
   d. endoderm

3. The corpus luteum acts as the placenta for the implanted ovum until
   a. the first gestational month
   b. the fifth gestational month
   c. the fourth gestational month
   d. the end of the second gestational month

4. A mother in the outpatient clinic stated to the nurse, "I'm sure I'm going to have a boy infant because my husband says he knows it's a boy." The correct response from the nurse would be which of the following?
   a. "You could be right."
   b. "The female determines the sex of the fetus."
   c. "There are more girls born than boys."
   d. "The male sex cell determines the sex of the child."

5. If a patient expelled a 25-cm fetus prematurely, what is the approximate gestational age of the fetus?
   a. 3 months
   b. 5 months
   c. 2 months
   d. 4 months

6. A fetal neural tube defect can be diagnosed as early as 16 weeks' gestation. Which of the following substances is examined to determine such abnormalities?
   a. estrogen
   b. progesterone
   c. alpha-fetoprotein
   d. luteinizing hormone

7. Amino acids are transferred through the uteroplacental blood flow by which of the following processes?
   a. capacitation
   b. active transport
   c. simple diffusion
   d. ustulation

8. A pregnant woman in the outpatient department asked the nurse what position she should lay so the baby would get the most oxygen. Which of the following is the best answer?
   a. "On your back with two pillows under your head."
   b. "On your left side."
   c. "On your right side."
   d. "It really doesn't matter."

9. A pregnant woman in the outpatient department shared with the nurse that she smoked and asked if she could continue to do so. The nurse's best response would be
   a. "How much do you smoke?"
   b. "You should probably decrease the number of cigarettes to ten a day."
   c. "Women who smoke usually have smaller babies than nonsmokers."
   d. "That is something you should ask the physician."

10. A pregnant woman in the outpatient clinic confided in the nurse that she has frequent headaches and has always taken aspirin. Which of the following would be the nurse's best response?
    a. "Do you remember if you took aspirin in the first 4 weeks of your pregnancy?"
    b. "The doctor may recommend another medication for your headaches."
    c. "Could you tell me more about these headaches and when you get them?"
    d. "We don't recommend any medication during pregnancy."

ANSWER KEY

1. *Correct response: b*
The fertilized ovum implants in the decidua.
  a. This is a germ layer.
  c and d. These structures form the placenta.
Knowledge/Physiologic/Assessment

2. *Correct response: a*
The ectoderm forms the fetal nervous system.
  b. The mesoderm forms muscles, bone, cartilage, teeth dentin, ligaments, tendons, kidneys, heart, and so forth.
  c. The entoderm forms the epithelium of digestive tract, epithelium of respiratory tract.
  d. This is another name for entoderm.
Knowledge/Physiologic/Assessment

3. *Correct response: d*
In the third month, placental function is operational.
  a, b, and c. These gestational months are incorrect.
Knowledge/Physiologic/Assessment

4. *Correct response: d*
The male sex cell determines a fetus's sex.
  a. This would be a nonprofessional response.
  b. This is an inappropriate statement.
  c. Although this statement is correct, it is not an appropriate response to the patient's question.
Comprehensive/Physiologic/Implementation

5. *Correct response: b*
The average fetal length at 5 months' gestation is 25 cm.
  a. 7 to 9 cm in length = 3 months.
  c. 2.5 cm in length = 2 months.
  d. 10 to 17 cm in length = 4 months.
Comprehensive/Physiologic/Assessment

6. *Correct response: c*
MSAFP screening can detect a fetus as risk for neural tube defects.

  a and b. Levels of these hormones increase throughout pregnancy; if they decrease, the woman will abort.
  d. Leutinizing hormone (LH) level has no bearing on fetal neural tube abnormalities.
Analysis/Physiologic/Analysis (Dx)

7. *Correct response: b*
Amino acids move through the placental barrier by way of active transport.
  a. Capacitation refers to penetration of the ovum by the sperm.
  c. An example of simple diffusion is oxygen transport to the fetus.
  d. Ustulation refers to the drying of a moist drug by heat.
Knowledge/Physiologic/NA

8. *Correct response: b*
Lying on the left side relieves pressure of the gravid uterus on the vena cava.
  a. With the woman supine with head elevated, the gravid uterus pushes against the diaphragm.
  c. With the woman lying on her right side, the gravid uterus pushes against the vena cava and decreases flow.
  d. This is an appropriate response.
Application/Physiologic/Implementation

9. *Correct response: c*
Smoking during pregnancy has been proven to increase the risk of a small-for-gestational age (SGA) infant.
  a and b. These responses may be helpful, but neither is the best response in this situation.
  d. The nurse can intervene independently of the physician in this situation.
Application/Physiologic/Implementation

10. *Correct response: c*
With this response, the nurse is probing to determine more about the cause of the headaches.
  a. During organogenesis, medications

can cause the greatest damage; this
response could cause worry.

b. This response does not address the
problem of the cause of the headaches.

d. This response is too restrictive.

Application/Physiologic/Implementation

Fertility and Infertility

I. Overview

A. Fertility

1. Male and female reproductive potential depend on multiple factors, including age, sex, and overall health status.
2. See Chapters 2 and 3 for further discussions of fertility and the processes of conception.

B. Infertility

1. Infertility is defined as the inability to conceive and carry a pregnancy to viability after at least 1 year of regular sexual intercourse without contraception.
2. Primary infertility: no previous history of either partner conceiving or impregnating
3. Secondary infertility: inability to conceive or carry to viability a pregnancy after previous successful pregnancy
4. Although infertility implies that some potential for conception exists, sterility denotes a total and irreversible inability to become pregnant or to impregnate.

C. **Incidence of infertility**
1. Involuntary childlessness is on the rise, with 15% to 20% of U.S. couples experiencing infertility.
2. Under optimum conditions, it is estimated that only about 25% of couples who try to conceive will do so within a month.
3. Female causes account for about 40% of all cases of infertility; male dysfunction accounts for another 40% of all cases of infertility, usually a sperm production problem.

D. **Etiology**
1. Causes of female infertility include:
   a. Vaginal causes (e.g., vaginal infections, anatomical abnormalities, sexual dysfunction that prevents penetration by the penis, a highly acidic vaginal environment, which markedly decreases sperm survival)
   b. Cervical causes, such as a disruption in any of the physiologic changes that normally occur during the preovulatory and ovulatory period that makes the cervical environment conducive to sperm survival (e.g., opening of the cervical os, increased alkalinity, increased secretions, ferning), and mechanical problems like cervical incompetence associated with women whose mothers were treated with diethylstilbestrol (DES) during pregnancy
   c. Uterine causes may be functional (e.g., an unfavorable environment for the travel of the sperm up the uterus into the fallopian tubes or for implantation after fertilization) or structural (e.g., uterine myomas or leiomyomas).
   d. Tubal causes are becoming more prominent with the increase incidence of pelvic inflammatory disease (PID), which leads to scarring that obstructs the fallopian tubes; the increased use of intrauterine devices (IUDs) contributes to the rise in PID, because 40% of infections associated with IUD use are asymptomatic and thus go untreated. Endometriosis also can contribute to tubal obstruction.
   e. Ovarian causes include anovulation, oligo-ovulation, and polycystic ovary syndrome; secretory malfunctions also contribute (e.g., inadequate progesterone secretion or an inadequate luteal phase will interfere with the ability for a fertilized ovum to be maintained).
2. Causes of male infertility include:
   a. Congenital factors (e.g., maternal history of DES ingestion during pregnancy, absence of the vasa deferentia or the testes)
   b. Ejaculation problems (e.g., retrograde ejaculation associated with diabetes, nerve damage, medications, or surgical trauma)

      c.   Sperm abnormalities (e.g., inadequate sperm production or maturation, inadequate motility, blockage of sperm along the male reproductive tract, or inability to deposit sperm in the vagina)

      d.   Testicular abnormalities due to illness (e.g., orchitis associated with mumps after puberty), cryptorchidism, trauma, or irradiation

      e.   Coital difficulties due to such causes as obesity or spinal nerve damage

      f.   Drugs (e.g., methotrexate, amebicides, sex hormones, and nitrofurantoin) that interfere with spermatogenesis

      g.   Other factors that interfere with sperm or semen production, including infections (e.g., sexually transmitted diseases), stress and inadequate nutrition, excessive alcohol intake, and nicotine

   3.   Interactive causes result from problems specific to the couple, such as:

      a.   Insufficient frequency of sexual intercourse

      b.   Poor timing of intercourse

      c.   Development of antibodies against a partner's sperm

II. Evaluation and diagnosis of infertility

A. Initial assessment

   1.   Evaluation of infertility begins with physical examination of both partners and basic laboratory tests including complete blood count, thyroid function tests, and urinalysis.

   2.   If these results are negative, an infertility work-up consisting of more intensive tests is begun.

B. Diagnostic studies

   1.   Semen analysis

      a.   Done after 48 to 72 hours of abstinence from orgasm to avoid false low readings

      b.   Repeated serial analysis is done 74 days apart

      c.   Sperm count, volume of ejaculate, presence of infection, semen viscosity, presence or absence of agglutination of sperm are considered

   2.   Postcoital test

      a.   Couple instructed to have sexual intercourse at the presumed time of ovulation, after a 48-hour period of abstinence

      b.   Within 8 hours of intercourse, a sample of cervical mucus is examined microscopically for characteristics that enhance sperm survival and for indications of adequate estrogen production.

   3.   Basal temperature recordings

      a.   Oral temperatures are taken daily by the woman before arising and recorded for several cycles.

       b.   A biphasic pattern with persistent temperature elevation for 12 to 14 days before menstruation is a favorable clinical finding.

   4.   Serum progesterone test or endometrial biopsy

       a.   A blood sample is drawn during the presumed luteal phase of the menstrual cycle.

       b.   An adequate amount of progesterone suggests that ovulation has probably occurred. (The normal serum progesterone level is 10 ng/mL or higher, with a lower level of 3 to 4 ng/mL at an earlier stage of the luteal phase.)

       c.   Endometrial biopsy provides direct histologic information about the endometrial tissue.

       d.   If adequate secretory tissue is seen, secretion of progesterone and luteinizing hormone is normal, thus indicating that ovulation has occurred.

   5.   Hysterosalpingography

       a.   Radiopaque dye is injected through the cervix into the uterus. Fluoroscopy shows whether the fallopian tubes fill with dye.

       b.   A radiograph is taken 24 hours later to determine if the dye has dispersed in the pelvic cavity, an indication of fallopian tube patency.

       c.   Must be done after menstruation has ceased in order to prevent the possibility of old menstrual blood being pushed into the tubes and causing infection

       d.   Must be done before ovulation to prevent pushing a fertilized ovum out through the fimbrial end of the tubes

   6.   Other tests

       a.   Immunoassay of semen and male or female serum to determine if antibody formation against the partner's sperm is a factor in infertility

       b.   Sperm penetration assay, an in vitro test to determine the ability of the sperm to penetrate the zona pellucida of the ova from superovulated hamsters

III. Medical management of infertility

  A. Fertilization techniques

     1.   In vitro fertilization

       a.   Used when damaged or obstructed fallopian tubes impair transport of a fertilized egg to the uterus

       b.   First recorded success in 1978 in England

       c.   Following a course of infertility drugs (e.g., Clomid, Pergonal) to stimulate ovulation, the ovary is punctured during laparoscopy and mature follicles are removed by suction.

       d.   Each egg is incubated for several hours in a sugar, salt, and protein mixture designed to simulate maternal fluids found in the fallopian tubes.

    e. Semen is added and the eggs and fluid are again incubated; if the egg is fertilized, it is incubated further until cell division begins, at which time the fertilized egg is deposited in the woman's uterus using a thin plastic catheter.

2. Surrogate embryo transfer (SET)

    a. Used in situations where the woman is not capable of producing normal mature mature follicles but where the male partner is fertile

    b. The first SET was born in 1984.

    c. Using hormonal therapy, the menstrual cycles of the donor and recipient women are synchronized.

    d. Sperm of the fertile spouse is artificially inseminated in the fertile donor following her normal ovulation.

    e. If fertilization occurs, several days later the fertilized egg is washed from the donor's uterus and deposited in the recipient's uterus; if successful, implantation occurs soon afterward.

3. Gamete intrafallopian transfer (GIFT)

    a. An ovum is surgically retrieved from the ovary and implanted into the fallopian tube.

    b. Sperm are then implanted into the fallopian tube.

    c. It is hoped that fertilization then occurs naturally.

4. In vivo fertilization or embryo transplantation

    a. Indicated when the recipient woman is unable to conceive naturally but can carry a fetus to maturity

    b. An embryo conceived in one woman is transplanted into the uterus of another.

    c. Genetically, the fetus is the result of the union of the male's sperm with the ovum of the donor woman.

5. Surrogate mothering

    a. Used when a woman is not only unable to conceive but also unable to carry a fetus to viability

    b. Semen from the partner is artificially inseminated into the host (surrogate mother).

    c. After birth, the infant is given to the infertile couple.

    d. Legislation is pending in many states to regulate this practice.

B. Other treatments

1. Medical interventions include:

    a. Altering acidic cervical mucus by having the woman douche with an alkaline solution ½ hour before intercourse

    b. Removing environmental hazards associated with oli-

gospermia (e.g., tight underclothes, hot tubs or saunas, certain drugs, chemicals, and toxins)
  2. Surgical interventions may include:
    a. Correction of anatomical defects and removal of obstructions in the female reproductive tract (e.g., removal of uterine fibroids, cerclage of an incompetent cervix, microsurgery to open blocked fallopian tubes)
    b. Ligation of varicocele in the male
  3. Pharmocologic interventions can include:
    a. Antibiotic therapy to treat infections
    b. Testosterone to treat oligospermia
    c. Estrogen therapy to increase the abundance of cervical mucus and enhance ferning and spinnbarkheit
    d. Ovulation-induction medications to treat anouvlation

C. **Sexual therapy**
  1. This therapy for infertility involves treatment of sexual problems that may interfere with conception (e.g., vaginismus or dyspareunia without an identifiable organic, physical, or mechanical cause; psychogenic impotence).
  2. One approach is sex counseling involving gathering assessment data on a couple's sexual difficulties, then clarifying each member's perceptions of the other and of sexual activities in general.
  3. The therapist facilitates communication between the two partners and their acceptance of each other's feelings and attitudes.
  4. The couple may be taught specific exercises and different coital positions to assist in increasing control during sexual activity or enjoyment in the pleasure of sex.

IV. **Implications for nursing**
  A. **Assessment**
    1. Evaluate the couple's sexual and reproductive history to rule out sexual dysfunction as a cause of infertility.
    2. Assess the couple's knowledge of sexuality, sexual techniques, and infertility.
    3. Perform a complete physical examination and arrange for appropriate diagnostic and laboratory tests for both partners.
    4. Also assess the couple's:
      a. General lifestyle, including use of medicines, drugs, and other substances; nutrition; exercise and rest patterns
      b. Usual strategies for coping with stress and anxiety
      c. Psychosocial responses associated with infertility—stage of emotional healing, cultural influences, belief systems, and effect on self-image

  B. **Nursing diagnoses**
    1. Ineffective Family/Individual Coping
    2. Knowledge Deficit

3. Self-concept Disturbance
4. Sexual Dysfunction
5. Spiritual Distress
C. Planning and implementation
   1. Keep in mind that diagnosis and treatment of infertility typically occurs over the course of several years and represents a significant financial and emotional commitment.
   2. Assist the couple to regain a sense of control by:
      a. Using stress reduction techniques
      b. Pointing out successes and achievements in other areas of their lives
   3. Provide support for decision-making and advocacy, including:
      a. Nonjudgmental listening and facilitation of decision-making
      b. Time to talk out ideas, concerns, issues of conflict
      c. Access to other sources and networks for information and support
      d. Referral to appropriate agencies
   5. Provide anticipatory guidance related to:
      a. The complex battery of diagnostic tests
      b. Protocols of fertility evaluation
      c. Responses to such procedures and the impact on sexual functioning and the couple's relationship
   6. Provide accurate information and dispel myths associated with infertility that foster guilt, self-doubt, and feelings of inadequacy.
   7. Help the couple resolve their feelings about infertility.
D. Evaluation
   1. The infertile couple demonstrates positive adjustment to the demands of the diagnostic and treatment regimens.
   2. The infertile partners verbalize their individual and collective feelings related to infertility, diagnosis, and treatment.
   3. The infertile couple exhibits evidence of healthy coping mechanisms in dealing with infertility.

Bibliography

Danforth, D. N. (Ed.). (1986). *Obstetrics and gynecology* (5th ed.). Philadelphia: J. B. Lippincott.

Jensen, M. D., & Bobak, I. M. (1985). *Maternity and gynecologic care: The nurse and family* (3rd ed.). St. Louis: C. V. Mosby.

May, K. A., & Mahlmeister, L. R. (1990). *Comprehensive maternity nursing: Nursing process and the childbearing family* (2nd ed.). Philadelphia: J. B. Lippincott.

Olds, S. (1984). *Maternity-newborn nursing*. Menlo Park, CA: Addison-Wesley.

Reeder, S. J., & Martin, L. L. (1987). *Maternity nursing: Family, newborn, and women's health care* (16th ed.). Philadelphia: J. B. Lippincott.

STUDY QUESTIONS

1. Bob and Mary Jones have been trying to conceive for 2 years. Their records reveal no physiologic problem that would prevent conception. The nurse provides them with information about optimum timing of intercourse to increase the likelihood of conception, including all of the following *except*
   a. Ovulation occurs about 15 days before the onset of the next menstrual cycle.
   b. An ovulated egg has a lifespan of 12 to 24 hours.
   c. The male's abstinence from ejaculation for 72 to 96 hours increases the likelihood of conception.
   d. Ejaculated sperm have a lifespan of 24 to 48 hours.

2. Tom and Tina Brown have one child, aged 10 years. They have been trying for several years to have another child. Their situation would be referred to as
   a. primary infertility
   b. secondary infertility
   c. irreversible infertility
   d. viable infertility

3. In assessing the adequacy of sperm for conception, which of the following is the single most useful criterion?
   a. sperm count
   b. sperm motility
   c. sperm maturity
   d. semen volume

4. Susan Saget has come to the infertility clinic for assistance in becoming pregnant. In taking Susan's medical history during assessment, the nurse discovers that Susan's mother took the drug diethylstilbestrol (DES) during her pregnancy with Susan. Which of the following would be the most accurate analysis of this information?
   a. It is of concern because maternal DES use is linked to increased incidence of pelvic inflammatory disease in female offspring.
   b. It is of concern because maternal DES use is linked to cervical incompetence in female offspring.
   c. It is of no concern because maternal DES use is not linked to any problems in offspring.
   d. It is of no concern because maternal DES is linked to problems in male, not female, offspring.

5. During assessment, the nurse discovers that the patient's medical history includes a ruptured appendix and resulting peritonitis. Why might these data be pertinent to the patient's infertility problems?
   a. Resulting scarring and adhesions may have created anatomic deformities or tubal blocking.
   b. The infection may have caused sterility.
   c. The appendix plays a role in tubal functioning.
   d. Surgical removal of the appendix likely severed her fallopian tubes.

6. Joe and Amy Kramer want to conceive a child and have been trying for 3 years without success. They have gone through the stresses and discomfort of many diagnostic procedures. When discussing their situation with the nurse, Amy states that all the couples their age that they know are having their second or third child, yet they "are so inadequate that we can't even produce one." Amy goes on to state that "with my luck, I'd probably have a defective baby anyway." Joe tries to comfort her, saying "It's probably all my fault." Based on this information, the most pertinent nursing diagnosis for Joe and Amy would be
   a. Fear related to the unknown
   b. Altered Comfort related to numerous diagnostic procedures
   c. Ineffective Family Coping related to infertility
   d. Self-concept Disturbance related to infertility

7. Kyle and Kim Avery have not been able to conceive during the 5 years of their marriage. They have never used contraception and usually have intercourse three to four times a week. Both independently express a high degree of sexual satisfaction. They practice some sexual experimentation with position, time, and location for intercourse and express particular pleasure with the use of additional lubrication with petroleum jelly. Kyle's sperm count is lower than normal, but other assessment data appear to be well within normal limits. Based on these data, the nurse's recommendation for potentially increasing fertility would include which of the following initially?
   a. Reduce frequency of intercourse to less than once a week.
   b. Encourage them to achieve greater consistency in how they perform intercourse.
   c. Instruct them to eliminate the additional lubrication.
   d. Clarify the validity of the degree of sexual satisfaction.

8. Introduction of radiopaque material into the uterus and fallopian tubes to assess tubal patency is known as
   a. uterotubal insufflation
   b. laparoscopy
   c. culdoscopy
   d. hysterosalpingography

9. Mark and Cindy Hulce have been through numerous diagnostic procedures, and have just been told that their infertility problem is serious; Mark has a low sperm count and Cindy has uterine fibroids causing tubal blockage. Mark begins laughing and shaking his head, then Cindy begins to laugh with Mark, saying, "Oh, we were so worried nothing could be done. We'll just take care of these two things and then we'll have a baby." The couple's initial reaction to the news of their fertility problems most likely indicates which of the following?
   a. Denial of the severity of the problem
   b. Covered anger with one another
   c. Joyful relief at the good news about nonseriousness of the problem
   d. Coping with a positive attitude

10. Desperately desiring children, Peter and Marta Thomas have spent the past 10 years subjecting themselves to numerous diagnostic procedures. Each has undergone corrective surgical procedures, and they have gone through marital therapy to help them cope adaptively with their anger and disappointment. Today they share with the nurse that they have decided to forgo any more tests or procedures and will now seek to adopt a child. While talking to the nurse, they are smiling and holding hands, and Peter says that he's "glad I'll never have to see this place [the infertility clinic] again." Based on this information, the nurse would most accurately evaluate their behavior as demonstrating
    a. Denial of their chance to have their own child
    b. Anger at the nurse and the clinic for wasting their time
    c. Apathy and resignation concerning their infertility problems
    d. Acceptance of their infertility

ANSWER KEY

1. *Correct response: c*
Abstinence normally has no effect on conception.
  a, b, and d. These statements are all accurate.
Comprehensive/Safe care/Implementation

2. *Correct response: b*
Because Tom and Tina have successfully conceived, their situation would be accurately described as secondary infertility.
  a. Primary infertility would apply if the couple had never conceived a child.
  c. No information in this scenario suggests irreversible infertility.
  d. This is not an appropriate term in reference to infertility.
Comprehensive/Physiologic/Analysis

3. *Correct response: b*
Although all of the factors listed are important, sperm motility is the single most significant criteria in assessing male fertility.
  a, c, and d. Sperm count, sperm maturity, and semen volume are all significant, but they are not as significant as sperm motility.
Knowledge/Physiologic/Assessment

4. *Correct response: b*
Maternal DES use has been linked to cervical abnormalities in female offspring.
  a, c, and d. These statements are all incorrect analyses of the situation.
Comprehensive/Safe care/Assessment

5. *Correct response: a*
Scarring and adhesions are possible given this patient's history.
  b and d. These problems are both highly unlikely.
  c. This is an untrue statement.
Application/Physiologic/Analysis (Dx)

6. *Correct response: d*
The data presented most strongly support self-concept issues as the couple's primary problem.
  a, b, and c. Although these diagnoses could apply to this couple, Self-concept Disturbance would be the primary diagnosis.
Application/Safe care/Analysis (Dx)

7. *Correct response: c*
Petroleum jelly and some water-soluble lubricants have been shown to be spermicidal.
  a. Reducing the frequency of intercourse will not increase the probability of conception.
  b and d. The information presented does not support that these are factors in this couple's inability to conceive.
Analysis/Safe care/Implementation

8. *Correct response: d*
Although all the responses listed are diagnostic procedures, only hysterosalpingography involves a radiopaque material.
  a, b, and c. None of these procedures uses radiopaque material.
Comprehensive/Safe care/Assessment

9. *Correct response: a*
Denial is a typical initial reaction to "bad news" that allows time for adjustment to the threatening situation.
  b. Although Mark and Cindy may be angry with one another, there are no data here to support this analysis.
  c and d. This situation involves neither joy nor positive feelings.
Analysis/Psychosocial/Analysis (Dx)

10. *Correct response: d*
Peter and Marta are demonstrating acceptance of their situation by taking steps to obtain children despite their infertility.
  a and b. This couple's history of 10 years of therapeutic assistance indicates that they have moved through denial and anger.
  c. They have not been apathetic and resigned but have made every effort to achieve conception.
Analysis/Psychosocial/Evaluation

Family Planning and Contraception

I. Overview

A. Family planning

1. Family planning is defined as the conscious process whereby a couple decides on the number and spacing of children and the timing of births.

2. Specific objectives of family planning include:

   a. Avoid unwanted pregnancies through contraception.

   b. Regulate intervals between pregnancies.

   c. Determine the number of children in the family.

   d. Control the time at which births occur.

   e. Facilitate wanted births for women with fertility problems.

   f. Prevent pregnancy for women with serious illness in whom pregnancy would pose a health risk.

   g. Provide the option of avoiding pregnancy to women who are carriers of genetic disease.

3. The overall goal of nursing intervention in family planning is to improve general maternal, neonatal, and family health.

4. Preconception planning—an ideal not always realized—provides an opportunity for the couple to enhance the probability of a healthy baby. It includes health history and physical examination of both partners and appropriate teaching relative to physical, psychological, and financial preparation for pregnancy and childbirth.

B. Nursing care

1. Defined as prevention of pregnancy, contraception can take many forms.

2. Knowledge of available contraceptive methods and their advantages and disadvantages is vital to nurses's role in reproductive health care in order to provide information.

3. To provide effective care, the nurse must understand and be comfortable talking about contraception and sexuality.

4. A thorough health assessment and history is essential to planning appropriate contraception teaching.

5. Choice of appropriate contraceptive method must consider many factors, including:
   a. Religious orientation
   b. Social and cultural values
   c. Medical contraindications
   d. Psychological contraindications

6. The best contraceptive method is one that is the most comfortable and natural for the partners and one that they will use correctly and consistently.

7. Contraceptive effectiveness is defined in terms of maximal effectiveness and typical effectiveness:
   a. Maximal effectiveness: conditions (i.e., when completely understood and used as recommended)
   b. Typical effectiveness: a method's effectiveness under actual use, in which some people use the method correctly and others use it carelessly or incorrectly

II. Contraceptive methods

  A. Natural or fertility awareness methods

1. Calendar method
   a. Calculated by subtracting 18 days from the end of the shortest cycle and subtracting 11 days from the end of the longest cycle to determine the fertile period
   b. 12 months of recorded menstrual cycles are needed to determine the longest and shortest cycles; continued recordings are necessary.
   c. Requires long periods of abstinence and correct calculations to be effective

        d.   Confusing irregular bleeding with a menstrual cycle can lead to incorrect calculations.

    2.   Basal body temperature (BBT) method

        a.   Uses the single sign of rise in BBT to predict ovulation

        b.   Temperature is taken orally or rectally each morning before rising.

        c.   BBT lowers before ovulation; BBT rises 0.4 to 0.8 degrees with ovulation in response to production of progesterone from the corpus luteum.

        d.   Abstinence begins the first day of menses and continues until the third day of temperature elevation.

        e.   Coitus is confined to the postovulatory period, usually about 10 days.

    3.   Cervical mucus method

        a.   Character, appearance, and amount of cervical mucus will change due to estrogen and progesterone.

        b.   Cervical mucus becomes clear, slippery (egg white consistency), and increases in quantity in response to high estrogen levels.

        c.   During preovulatory and postovulatory periods, mucus is yellowish, decreases in quantity, and becomes thick and sticky, inhibiting sperm movement.

    4.   Symptothermal method

        a.   Combination of the above techniques for determining the fertile period

        b.   Provides couple with more information; more complex and difficult to learn

    5.   Natural methods are indicated for couples motivated to spend time and effort learning how to control their own fertility or when other methods are not appropriate due to medical, religious, or personal preference.

    6.   These methods are contraindicated in infertility.

    7.   Advantages: free or inexpensive, no untoward effects; encourages couple communication; these techniques are noncontroversial and may be included in sex education programs.

    8.   Disadvantages: takes a great deal of self-control to be effective; disruptive in that they require regular abstinence for a specific number of days; relies on signs and symptoms of fertility, which may not be easily detected.

    9.   Effectiveness is variable, depending on individual and couple discipline.

B. **Coitus interruptus**

    1.   Withdrawal of the penis from the vagina before ejaculation occurs

    2.   No indications or contraindications except personal preference

    3.   Advantages: no expense, medically safe

       4.   Disadvantages: high incidence of pregnancy; interruption of sexual excitement or plateau

       5.   Effectiveness: ineffective because there are sperm in pre-ejaculate fluid and because there tends to be diminished pleasure for both partners

C. Spermicides

       1.   Substances that interfere with viability of sperm and prevent sperm from entering the cervix

       2.   Indicated when other methods cannot be used; contraindicated with vaginal tissue irritation from alum

       3.   Disadvantages: low effectiveness and aesthetically unpleasant

       4.   Advantages: available in jellies, creams, suppositories, and foams; available without prescription with no serious side effects

       5.   Must be applied within 30 minutes before intercourse and reapplied before each subsequent coitus; no douching for 8 hours after intercourse

D. Sponge

       1.   Vaginal contraceptive sponge with central dimple that fits over the cervix, made of polyurethane and contains spermicide

       2.   No indications or contraindications

       3.   Disadvantages: must be soaked in water before use; unwanted pregnancies have occurred; because it covers the cervix, there is a tendency toward vaginal dryness and subsequent infection (e.g., toxic shock syndrome).

       4.   Advantages: can be left in place 24 to 30 hours; can be used for multiple coitus

       5.   Side effects and complications include difficulty removing, pregnancy, allergic reactions, vaginal dryness, and toxic shock syndrome.

E. Condom

       1.   A rubber sheath applied over the penis after erection, providing a mechanical barrier to prevent sperm from entering vagina

       2.   Indicated when other methods cannot be used

       3.   Disadvantages: vaginal jelly should be used if condom or vagina is dry; may cause a decrease in sensation for some couples

       4.   Advantages: helps prevent venereal disease; available without prescription; no serious side effects

F. Cervical cap

       1.   A small rubber or plastic dome that fits snugly over the cervix

       2.   Advantages: plastic cap can be left in place 3 to 4 weeks; rubber cap can be left in place 24 to 36 hours; valvular cap (not currently available in United States) may be left in place up to 1 year.

       3.   Disadvantages: must be used in conjunction with spermicidal gel or cream in the cap

       4.   Indicated when other methods cannot be used

5. Contraindicated in the presence of anatomic abnormalities, or with allergies to rubber, plastic, or spermicide
6. Side effects and complications include trauma to cervix or vagina, interference with menstrual flow and with flow of cervical mucus, pelvic infection, cervicitis, abnormal Pap test.
7. Effectiveness is increased when used with spermicide.

G. Diaphragm

1. Flexible ring covered with a dome-shaped rubber cap that is inserted into the vagina to cover the cervix
2. Must be used with spermicidal jelly or cream placed in the center of dome and around the rim; the patient is instructed to insert the diaphragm no more than 2 hours before intercourse and leave it in place for 6 hours after coitus; additional spermicide is needed if intercourse is repeated, taking care not to dislodge the diaphragm.
3. Must be refitted after childbirth or if there has been a weight loss of 15 lb
4. Side effects and complications include toxic shock syndrome, cystitis, cramps or rectal pressure, and allergic reaction to spermicide or rubber.

H. Intrauterine device (IUD)

1. Flexible device that is inserted into the uterine cavity, where it causes a localized sterile inflammatory reaction
2. Effectiveness: 97% maximum and 93% typical
3. Inexpensive form of contraception, because once inserted it requires no attention other than to determine that it is still in place
4. Contraindications include pregnancy, active or chronic pelvic infection, postpartum infection, endometrial hyperplasia or carcinoma, abnormalities of uterus.
5. Side effects include dysmenorrhea, increased menstrual flow, spotting between periods.
6. Complications include uterine infection, uterine perforation, and ectopic pregnancy.
7. Danger signs include late or missed menstrual period; severe abdominal pain; temperature and chills; foul-smelling vaginal discharge; and spotting, bleeding, or heavy menstrual periods.

I. Oral contraceptives

1. Combination estrogen and progesterone preparation in pill form; estrogen and progesterone inhibit the release of follicle-stimulating hormone and luteinizing hormone and release of an ovum.
2. Indicated when the most effective contraceptive method other than sterilization is desired
3. Contraindications include pregnancy, history of thrombophlebitis, circulatory disease, varicosities, diabetes, estrogen-dependent carcinomas, liver disease, heavy smoking, or age over 35 years.

4. Side effects include breakthrough bleeding, nausea, vomiting, susceptibility to vaginal infections, thrombus formation, edema, weight gain, irritability, or missed periods.
5. Numerous oral contraceptives are available, with differing hormones and hormone combinations.
6. Biphasic and triphasic contraceptives closely mirror the hormonal fluctuations for the menstrual cycle.
7. Reassessment and evaluation is essential every 6 months; danger signals include abdominal pain, chest pain or shortness of breath, headaches, blurred or loss of vision, leg pain in calf or thigh.

J. Sterilization
1. Vasectomy (male): surgical ligation of the vas deferens, which terminates passage of sperm through vas; sterilization compete once male reproductive tract cleared of spermatozoa; reversal success varies: anatomical, 40% to 90%; clinical, 18% to 60%
2. Tubal ligation (female): surgical ligation or cauterization of fallopian tubes; possible reversal by reconstruction of tubes: success rate, 50% to 70%
3. These procedures are indicated when pregnancies are not desired for medical or personal reasons; the finality of sterilization should be stressed.
4. Advantages and disadvantages: in most instances, these are permanent, nonreversible procedures.

III. Implications for nursing
A. Assessment
1. Determine the type of contraception the woman or couple desires.
2. Obtain a thorough medical, surgical, menstrual, and obstetrical history to identify any contraindications to the desired method.
3. Perform a precontraception physical examination to include breast and pelvic examination, vital sign measurement, and other aspects as appropriate.
4. Arrange for and evaluate results of appropriate precontraception laboratory tests (e.g., Pap smear, serologic test for syphilis, culture for gonorrhea, urinalysis, and complete blood count).

B. Nursing diagnoses
1. Altered Health Maintenance
2. Knowledge Deficit
3. Self-care Deficit

C. Planning and implementation
1. Evaluate the woman's or couple's knowledge of available methods; provide information to correct misconceptions.
2. Assist the woman or couple in choosing an appropriate method.
3. Teach the woman or couple about the chosen method, including, as appropriate:

        a.   Insertion and removal (e.g., diaphragm)
        b.   Application and removal (e.g., condom)
        c.   Dosage schedule for oral contraceptives
        d.   Techniques for natural methods
    4.   Discuss possible side effects and steps to take if they occur.

D.   **Evaluation**

    1.   The woman or couple verbalizes satisfaction with the selected contraceptive method.

    2.   The woman or couple demonstrates accurate understanding of how to use the selected method.

    3.   The woman or couple verbalizes any danger signs associated with the method selected.

Bibliography

Danforth, D. N. (Ed.). (1986). *Obstetrics and gynecology* (5th ed.). Philadelphia: J. B. Lippincott.

Jensen, M. D., & Bobak, I. M. (1985). *Maternity and gynecologic care: The nurse and family* (3rd ed.). St. Louis: C. V. Mosby.

May, K. A., & Mahlmeister, L. R. (1990). *Comprehensive maternity nursing: Nursing process and the childbearing family* (2nd ed.). Philadelphia: J. B. Lippincott.

Olds, S. (1984). *Maternity-newborn nursing*. Menlo Park, CA: Addison-Wesley.

Reeder, S. J., & Martin, L. L. (1987). *Maternity nursing: Family, newborn, and women's health care* (16th ed.). Philadelphia: J. B. Lippincott.

STUDY QUESTIONS

1. The nurse would instruct a breast-feed-ing woman to use which of the follow-ing contraceptive methods?
   a. birth control pills
   b. estrogen injections
   c. IUD
   d. condom and spermicidal foam com-bination

2. Which of the following would likely be the *least* effective means of contraception for most couples?
   a. temperature thermal-calendar method
   b. intrauterine device
   c. spermicidal jelly or cream
   d. douching after intercourse

3. The most effective spermicidal contra-ceptive agent generally is
   a. spermicidal cream
   b. spermicidal jelly
   c. spermicidal foam
   d. spermicidal vaginal suppository

4. The IUD prevents pregnancy by which of the following mechanisms?
   a. altering the environment in the fal-lopian tubes
   b. altering the environment in the en-dometrium
   c. altering the speed at which the ovum travels
   d. through an unclear mechanism

5. Natural family planning involves avoid-ing artificial methods to prevent preg-nancy and relying on normal physiologic practices. Which one of the following best describes natural family planning?
   a. the calendar method
   b. temperature thermal and calendar method
   c. the Billing's and temperature thermal method
   d. the temperature method

6. When counseling a patient about contra-ceptive methods, the nurse would specify that the most effective means of contracep-tion generally is considered to be
   a. spermicidal jelly or cream

   b. IUD
   c. rhythm-Billing method
   d. postcoital douche

7. When advising a 35-year-old woman who delivered her third child and smokes one pack of cigarettes per day, the nurse most likely would promote which of the following contraceptive methods?
   a. the sponge
   b. birth control pills
   c. sterilization
   d. IUD

8. A postpartum teenaged mother confides to the nurse that she "will never get pregnant again because I'll never have sex again." Which of the following would be the nurse's best response to this statement?
   a. "That's a good decision and I ap-prove of it."
   b. "Usually teens who have had sexual experience want to continue sexual experience."
   c. "You may want to be in control of what happens to you in the future, so contraceptive practice may be a good plan."
   d. "If your school has a sex education course, you should enroll in it."

9. For a woman using a diaphragm for con-traception, the nurse should advise her to leave the device in place for how long after intercourse?
   a. 1 hour
   b. 12 hours
   c. 28 hours
   d. 6 hours

10. Most women can use the same dia-phragm for years if proper care is main-tained. But which of the following situa-tions would warrant remeasurement and possibly a refitting?
    a. weight gain or loss of 5 lb
    b. surgery involving general anesthetic
    c. surgery involving regional anesthesia
    d. pelvic surgery

ANSWER KEY

1. *Correct response: d*
   The condom and spermicidal foam combination is safest for a breast-feeding infant.
   a and b. Estrogen and progesterone cross over into breast milk.
   c. A woman can resume intercourse prior to 6 weeks after delivery, but an IUD or diaphragm cannot be fitted until 6 weeks after delivery.
   Application/Safe care/Planning

2. *Correct response: d*
   Douching can force sperm through the cervix, possibly facilitating fertilization.
   a. Although this method is not considered very effective, it is more effective than douching.
   b. An IUD is a very effective contraceptive method.
   c. Spermicidal jelly or cream is not as statistically effective as some other methods.
   Comprehensive/Health promotion/Planning

3. *Correct response: c*
   The aerosol property of foam makes it more effective because it can disperse more effectively to cover the cervix.
   a. The cream may have the same chemical properties; however, it melts at body temperature.
   b. Jelly does not melt like cream; however, it does not disperse, as does foam.
   d. Suppositories do foam when inserted into vaginal secretions; however, this action is not similar to the aerosol action.
   Comprehensive/Health promotion/Planning

4. *Correct response: b*
   The IUD acts as a foreign body and sets up a foreign body reaction or low-grade inflammation, which prevents implantation of a fertilized ovum.
   a and c. These mechanisms are not known to occur.

   d. The mechanism is known (a foreign body reaction).
   Analysis/Physiologic/Analysis (Dx)

5. *Correct response: c*
   The Billing's method checks for thickness and stretchability of the cervical secretions after ovulation, and the temperature thermal method checks for an elevation of temperature after progesterone stimulation (ovulation).
   a. This method alone is not effective.
   b. These methods are the same.
   d. This method alone is not optimum.
   Analysis/Physiologic/Assessment

6. *Correct response: b*
   Of those methods listed, an IUD is the most effective.
   a. Spermicides are effective, but not as effective as an IUD.
   c. Natural methods can be effective only for women with regular menstrual cycles; even then, effectiveness is not great.
   d. Douching is the most ineffective of the four methods.
   Analysis/Health promotion/Planning

7. *Correct response: d*
   Of the methods listed, the IUD is the most effective except for sterilization.
   a. The sponge is not very effective for women who have had several children.
   b. Oral contraceptives are not given to older women who smoke because of the risk of embolism.
   c. The nurse would not recommend sterilization because of its permanency.
   Analysis/Safe care/Planning

8. *Correct response: c*
   Research has demonstrated that adolescents respond better to contraceptive teaching when they believe that they are in control.
   a. This is a judgmental response.
   b. This is true, as proven by research.

d. This an inappropriate response.
Analysis/Health promotion/Implementation

9. *Correct response: d*

The diaphragm should remain in place 6 hours after each (if applicable) subsequent intercourse.

a. After 1 hour, sperm will often be alive and able to permeate the cervix and fertilize the ovum.

b and c. This is too long for diaphragm retention and would predispose to infection.

Analysis/Safe care/Implementation

10. *Correct response: d*

Pelvic surgery can change the shape or size of pelvic structures, possibly requiring diaphragm refitting.

a. A weight gain or loss of 10 lb or more is the benchmark indicating the need for refitting.

b and c. Anesthesia does not have anything to do with anatomical changes of the pelvis.

Analysis/Health promotion/Implementation

Biopsychosocial Aspects
of Pregnancy

I. Biophysical changes in pregnancy

A. Overview

1. All maternal body systems are altered by pregnancy.
2. Such changes are normal, inevitable, and temporary.

B. Signs and symptoms of pregnancy

1. Presumptive (subjective) changes include:
   a. Amenorrhea
   b. Nausea and vomiting
   c. Urinary frequency
   d. Breast tenderness and changes

       e.   Excessive fatigue

2. Probable (objective) changes include:

   a.   Changes in pelvic organs:

     (1)   Goodell's sign: softening of the cervix

     (2)   Hegar's sign: softening of isthmus of uterus

     (3)   Ladin's sign: soft spot anteriorly in middle of the uterus

     (4)   McDonald's sign: flexibility of the uterus against the cervix

     (5)   Braun von Fernwald's sign: irregular, soft, enlarged area at the site of implantation

     (6)   Piskacek's sign: enlargement and softening of the uterus

   b.   Enlargement of abdomen

   c.   Uterine souffle (soft blowing sound at rate of maternal pulse)

   d.   Changes in skin pigmentation

   e.   Quickening (maternal perception of fetal movement)

3. Positive (diagnostic) changes include:

   a.   Fetal heart beat: audible at 10 to 12 weeks' gestation by Doppler and 16 to 20 weeks' gestation with a fetoscope; normal fetal heart rate is 120 to 160 beats per minute

   b.   Fetal movements palpable by examiner

   c.   Ultrasonography confirming presence of fetus

   d.   Fetal electrocardiography recording fetal heart pattern

C. **Reproductive system changes**

  1. Uterus

   a.   Uterine growth:

     (1)   Length: from 2½ inches to 12½ inches

     (2)   Width: from 1½ inches to 9½ inches

     (3)   Depth: from 1 inch to 8½ inches

     (4)   Weight: from 2½ oz to 2½ lb

     (5)   Volume: from 1 to 2 mL to 5000 mL

   b.   Enlargement results from increasing size of myometrial cells.

   c.   Hyperplasia of uterine muscle fibers occurs in the first 6 weeks of pregnancy. Hypertrophy of uterine muscle fibers and dilation of uterine blood vessels causes uterine enlargement after the first trimester.

   d.   Increased fibrous tissue adds strength and elasticity to the uterine muscle wall.

   e.   Uterine circulatory requirements increase; accordingly, so do the size and number of blood vessels and lymphatics.

   f.   Braxton Hicks contractions (painless contractions) occur intermittently throughout pregnancy and can be felt by the mother by the fourth month.

g. Normal uterine growth—measured in terms of fundal height—is evaluated in relation to other anatomic structures. After 20 weeks' gestation, fundal height in centimeters approximates the weeks of pregnancy.

2. Cervix
   a. Glandular tissue stimulated by estrogen
   b. Endocervical glands secrete thick mucus that forms a mucous plug
   c. The mucous plug seals the endocervical canal and prevents contamination of uterus by bacteria and other substances.
   d. The mucous plug is expelled when cervix begins to dilate.
   e. Goodell's sign (softening of the cervix) results from increased cervical vascularization.

3. Ovaries
   a. Do not produce ova during pregnancy
   b. Corpus luteum, which develops from ruptured follicle, produces hormones (estrogen and progesterone) for 10 to 12 weeks of pregnancy, then regresses by mid-pregnancy.

4. Vagina and external genitalia
   a. Increased vascularization causes tissue to thicken and soften.
   b. Increased vascularization of vagina causes a blue-purple coloration (Chadwick's sign).
   c. Vaginal discharges tends to be thick, white, and acidic (pH, 3.5 to 6.0).

5. Breasts
   a. Breast size increases and breast becomes more nodular due to glandular hyperplasia and hypertrophy.
   b. The nipple and areola become darker in color, with more prominent superficial veins.
   c. Striae may develop in late pregnancy.
   d. Colostrum may leak or be expressed from the breast during the last 3 months of pregnancy.

D. **Respiratory system changes**
   1. The diaphragm elevates and substernal angle increases due to an enlarging uterus.
   2. Displacement of diaphragm causes shortness of breath.
   3. Nasal stuffiness and epistaxis are common due to edema and vascular congestion induced by increased estrogen.
   4. Respiratory rate increases by about two breaths per minute and vital capacity increases slightly; breathing more deeply increases the efficiency of gas exchange. However, functional residual capacity and residual volume of air are decreased due to elevation of diaphragm.

E. **Cardiovascular system changes**
   1. Heart displaced upward, to the left, and forward

2. Blood volume increases 45% during pregnancy; red blood cell volume increases 20% to 30%; hematocrit decreases 7%, causing physiologic anemia of pregnancy; fibrin level may increase as much as 40%; leukocytes increase.
3. Pulse rate increases 10 to 15 beats per minute.
4. Blood pressure decreases slightly, then returns to near normal during the third trimester.
5. Supine hypotensive syndrome during the second trimester may be caused by pressure of enlarged uterus on the vena cava when the woman lies supine on her left side.

F. Gastrointestinal system changes
1. Nausea and vomiting frequently occur during the first trimester.
2. Gum tissue may become soft and bleed when traumatized.
3. Secretion of saliva may increase.
4. Gastric acidity decreases. Heartburn and flatulence often occur due to the reduction in gastric acidity, growing uterus, and smooth muscle relaxation.
5. Bloating and constipation may occur due to delayed gastric emptying time and decreased intestinal motility.

G. Urinary system changes
1. Urine output increases; urine-specific gravity decreases.
2. Dilatation of the kidneys and urethra may occur, especially on the right side, due to the pressure of the enlarged uterus.
3. Stasis of urine and urinary tract infection may occur due to dilated uterus.
4. The woman is at increased risk for glycosuria.
5. Urinary frequency occurs in the first and third trimesters due to pressure from the enlarged uterus.

H. Integumentary system changes
1. Pigmentation changes occur in the areola, nipple, vulva, perianal area, and linea alba.
2. Facial chloasma (mask of pregnancy) and vascular spider nevi may develop.
3. Striae (stretch marks) commonly appear on the abdomen, breasts, and thighs.
4. Activity of sebaceous and sweat glands may increase.

I. Skeletal system changes
1. Sacroiliac, sacrococcygeal, and pubic joints relax during pregnancy.
2. Symphysis pubis may separate slightly.
3. Lumbodorsal spinal curve is increased during the third trimester, commonly producing low back pain.

J. Metabolic changes
1. Metabolism accelerates during pregnancy.
2. Average weight gain is 24 to 30 lb, comprised of:

a. Fetus: 7½ lb
b. Placenta and membrane: 1½ lb
c. Amniotic fluid: 2 lb
d. Uterus: 2½ lb
e. Breasts: 3 lb
f. Increased blood volume: 2 to 4 lb
g. Extravascular fluid and fat: 4 to 9 lb

3. Water retention, about 7 L, commonly occurs during pregnancy.
   a. Fetus, placenta, and amniotic fluid: 3.5 L
   b. Increased blood volume, interstitial fluid, and hypertrophied maternal organs: 3.5 L

K. Endocrine system changes

1. Thyroid: increase in vascularity and hyperplasia; rise in thyroxin (T4), and 25% increase in basal metabolism rate
2. Parathyroid: concentration of hormone secreted and size of gland increases.
3. Pituitary
   a. Slight hypertrophy during pregnancy
   b. Anterior pituitary: prolactin responsible for beginning lactation after delivery
   c. Posterior pituitary: releases oxytocin (to produce uterine contractions) and vasopressin (to promote vasoconstriction and antidiuretic effect)
4. Adrenals: little structural change; cortisol levels regulate metabolism of carbohydrates and proteins.
5. Pancreas: increased insulin production
6. Placenta
   a. Endocrine gland of pregnancy
   b. Secretes human chorionic gonadotropin (HCG), estrogen, and progesterone
7. Hormones of pregnancy
   a. HCG: produced by the chorion, stimulates corpus luteum to produce estrogen and progesterone
   b. Human placental lactogen: increases circulating free fatty acids for maternal metabolism
   c. Estrogen: stimulates development of uterine environment for fetus (increases uterus in size and weight and augments blood supply)
   d. Progesterone: maintains endometrium and decreases contractility of the uterus
   e. Relaxin: decreases uterine activity and softens the cervix

L. Nutrition during pregnancy

1. Hormonal effects on nutrition stem from:
   a. Progesterone: causes relaxation of the smooth muscle, including the gastrointestinal tract, which reduces motility,

allowing more nutrients to be absorbed; increases maternal fat deposition; increases renal sodium excretion
   b. Estrogen: increases water retention
   c. HCG: implicated in morning nausea
2. Some metabolic adjustments during pregnancy are the basis for the increased nutritional requirements and dietary allowances. These include:
   a. A 50% greater plasma volume by 34 weeks' gestation than at conception, creating an increased need to carry oxygen and nutrients
   b. Increased serum lipid levels (triglycerides, cholesterol, free fatty acids, and vitamin A), probably due to increased circulating steroids, because cholesterol is a precursor for the synthesis of progesterone and estrogen in the placenta
   c. Increased blood flow through the kidneys and increased glomerular filtration rate to facilitate the clearance of waste products from mother and baby
3. The total energy cost of pregnancy is 80,000 calories; averaged over the entire pregnancy, it amounts to about 300 extra calories per day.
4. Protein requirements increase to provide sufficient amino acids for fetal development, increased blood volume, breast and uterine tissue growth; the recommended daily allowance is 30 g/day over nonpregnant needs (Table 6–1).
5. Pregnancy increases requirements for all vitamins.
6. Commonly recommended nutritional supplements contain vitamins B6, D, E, and C; folic acid, pantothenic acid, iron, calcium, magnesium, zinc, and copper.
7. Dietary calcium is the best way to increase calcium intake to support the growing fetus (e.g., dairy products, beans, leafy green vegetables [collard, mustard, kale, turnip, broccoli]).
8. Because of the mixed effects of calcium on iron and zinc absorption, daily calcium supplements > 100 g are not recommended during pregnancy.

TABLE 6–1.
Calorie, Protein, and Vitamin Requirements During Pregnancy

AGE IN YEARS	CALORIC REQUIREMENT (kcal/day)	PROTEIN REQUIREMENT (g/day)	FAT-SOLUBLE VITAMINS		
			A (μg/E)	D (μg)	E (mg TE)
11–14	2500	76	1000	15.0	10
15–18	2400	76	1000	15.0	10
19–22	2400	76	1000	12.5	10
23–50	2300	74	1000	10.0	10

        9.   Vitamin oversupplementation may lead to vitamin toxicity.

II. Psychosocial changes in pregnancy

A. Overview

1. Pregnant women tend to become more dependent, needing increased nurturing so they in turn can nurture their developing offspring.
2. Pregnant women need social service programs.

B. Psychosocial stages

1. Anticipatory stage—train for role; interact with other children
2. Honeymoon stage—full assumption of role; initially may need help from family members
3. Plateau stage—role fully exercised—either adequate or inadequate; may take several weeks, often about the time the mother resumes employment
4. Disengagement—termination stage, precedes and includes termination of the role; role of parenthood unclear as to when authority and obligation end

C. Meaning and effect of pregnancy on couple

1. The male partner experiences changes in perceived body space from the eighth month of gestation through the third postpartum month.
2. Men also may experience physical and psychological changes during their partner's pregnancy.
3. The coming child represents the synthesis of three distinct entities:
   a. Relationship of mother and partner
   b. Relationship of mother and the developing fetus
   c. Relationship of mother and the unique individual, the child
4. The mother can never again be a single unit.
5. Necessary tasks of pregnancy for a woman or couple include:
   a. Belief that she is pregnant and incorporation of fetus into body image
   b. Preparation for physical separation with birth of infant
   c. Resolution and identification of confusions that accompany role transition, thus preparing for smooth functioning of family
6. Common emotional reactions to pregnancy include:
   a. First trimester: ambivalence, fears, fantasies, anxiety
   b. Second trimester: feelings of well-being, increased need to learn about fetal growth and development; becomes narcissistic, passive, introverted; may seem egocentric and self-centered
   c. Third trimester: feels awkward, clumsy, not pretty; becomes more introverted; reflects on own childhood

III. Implications for nursing (Note: Also see Chapter 8, Antepartal Care)

A. Assessment

1. Initiate biopsychosocial assessment at the initial prenatal visit.
2. Perform ongoing data collection at each subsequent visit.
3. Make every effort to include the expectant father in the early prenatal visits.
4. Focus assessment on the expectant mother's and father's adaptation to pregnancy.
5. Evaluate for risk factors associated with poor adaptation:
   a. Prior negative childbearing or childrearing experiences
   b. Inadequate preparation for childbearing or childrearing
   c. Significant health concerns
   d. Negative response to the pregnancy
   e. Conflicts or problems in support system

B. Nursing diagnoses

1. Anxiety
2. Ineffective Family/Individual Coping
3. Altered Family Processes
4. Fear
5. Knowledge Deficit
6. Altered Role Performance
7. Self-concept Disturbance

C. Planning and implementation

1. Plan time to answer questions and concerns of both expectant parents.
2. Provide opportunities for ongoing psychosocial and biophysical assessment.
3. Teach effective self-care measures, as needed.
4. Provide anticipatory guidance (e.g., reassuring mother that nausea usually decreases, helping father understand that many men do not feel involved in the pregnancy until the last few weeks, explaining what to expect next month).

D. Evaluation

1. Expectant parents exhibit progress toward healthy adaptation to childbearing.
2. Expectant parents express satisfaction with increased knowledge level.

Bibliography

Danforth, D. N. (Ed.). (1986). *Obstetrics and gynecology* (5th ed.). Philadelphia: J. B. Lippincott.

Jensen, M. D., & Bobak, I. M. (1985). *Maternity and gynecologic care: The nurse and family* (3rd ed.). St. Louis: C. V. Mosby.

May, K. A., & Mahlmeister, L. R. (1990). *Comprehensive maternity nursing: Nursing process and the childbearing family* (2nd ed.). Philadelphia: J. B. Lippincott.

Olds, S. (1984). *Maternity-newborn nursing.* Menlo Park, CA: Addison-Wesley.

Reeder, S. J., & Martin, L. L. (1987). *Maternity nursing: Family, newborn, and women's health care* (16th ed.). Philadelphia: J. B. Lippincott.

STUDY QUESTIONS

1. The kidneys, ureter, and bladder change in structure and function during pregnancy. Which of the following is most frequently noted by the woman in the first trimester?
   a. dilation of the kidneys and ureters
   b. pressure and irritation of the bladder
   c. increased glomerular filtration rate
   d. urinary stasis

2. Gastrointestinal discomfort is common in the second trimester, most likely due to
   a. increased plasma HCG levels
   b. increased gastric emptying time
   c. pressure of the growing uterus and smooth muscle relaxation
   d. elevated estrogen levels

3. Chloasma, affecting approximately 70% of women during pregnancy, involves an irregular hyperpigmented area on the
   a. breasts
   b. chest, neck, arms, and legs
   c. abdomen, breast, and thighs
   d. cheeks, forehead, and nose

4. A pregnant patient states that she "waddles" when she walks. The nurse would explain that this is due to
   a. the large size of the baby
   b. pressure on the muscles
   c. relaxation of the pelvic joints
   d. excessive weight gain

5. The pregnant patient also says that a friend told her that weight gain during pregnancy shouldn't exceed 22 lb. The nurse should explain that optimum weight gain during pregnancy is
   a. 12 to 22 lb
   b. 15 to 25 lb
   c. 24 to 30 lb
   d. 25 to 40 lb

6. At 5 months' gestation, Sally West reports that she has felt intermittent painless contractions of her uterus, and asks the nurse about them. What would be the nurse's best response?
   a. "It is important to time these contractions, because it may be the beginning of labor."
   b. "If these contractions occur again, call your doctor immediately."
   c. "The contractions are Braxton Hicks contractions and they help increase the size of the uterus."
   d. "The contractions help stimulate the movement of blood through the placenta."

7. To a patient complaining of aching, swollen leg veins, the nurse would explain that this is most likely due to
   a. thrombophlebitis
   b. pregnancy-induced hypertension
   c. pressure against the veins in the pelvis
   d. force of gravity

8. During a prenatal visit, the nurse was able to feel fetal movements and auscultate the fetal heart rate with a fetoscope. These changes of pregnancy are known as
   a. expected changes
   b. presumptive changes
   c. probable changes
   d. positive changes

9. Women experience probable or objective changes during pregnancy—known as *probable* signs of pregnancy. Which one of the following is *not* a probable sign of pregnancy?
   a. Goodall's sign
   b. nausea
   c. changes in skin pigmentation
   d. positive pregnancy test

10. A pregnant woman experiences and accomplishes various psychosocial tasks of pregnancy. One of the first tasks she must accomplish is the acceptance of
    a. the infant by others
    b. the fetus as part of self
    c. safe passage through labor and delivery
    d. the infant's gender

ANSWER KEY

1. **Correct response: b**
   Pressure and irritation of the bladder result from the growing uterus.
   a and c. These occur in early pregnancy but are not noted by the woman.
   d. This can be a result of dilation of kidneys and ureters.
   Comprehensive/Physiologic/Analysis (Dx)

2. **Correct response: c**
   During the second trimester, pressure from the growing uterus and smooth muscle relaxation can cause GI discomfort.
   a. Increased HCG levels are present in the first trimester.
   b. Gastric emptying time is decreased in the second trimester.
   d. Estrogen levels are decreased in the second trimester.
   Comprehensive/Physiologic/Analysis (Dx)

3. **Correct response: d**
   Chloasma is marked by hyperpigmented areas on the face.
   a, b, and c. Chloasma is not seen on any of these areas.
   Knowledge/Safe care/Assessment

4. **Correct response: c**
   Pelvic relaxation due to hormonal changes can cause a waddling gait.
   a. The growing fetus will cause changes in posture.
   b. A growing uterus will produce pressure on muscles and cause discomfort.
   d. Weight gain will not affect the gait.
   Comprehensive/Physiologic/Evaluation

5. **Correct response: c**
   Normal weight gain during pregnancy ranges from 24 to 30 lb.
   a. This is insufficient weight gain.
   b. This is insufficient to marginally sufficient weight gain.
   d. This is excessive weight gain.
   Knowledge/Health promotion/
   Implementation

6. **Correct response: d**
   Braxton Hicks contractions are a normal antepartal phenomenon that stimulate placental perfusion.
   a. Braxton Hicks contractions are not a sign of labor.
   b. These contractions are normal and do not warrant notifying the physician.
   c. These contractions have no effect on uterine size.
   Application/Health promotion/
   Implementation

7. **Correct response: c**
   Pressure of the growing uterus will cause increased tendency toward blood stagnation in the lower extremities, resulting in edema and varicose vein formation.
   a. Thrombophlebitis is inflammation of veins due to thrombus formation.
   b. Pregnancy-induced hypertension is not associated with this complaint.
   d. Gravity is only a minor factor associated with this complaint.
   Application/Physiologic/Evaluation

8. **Correct response: d**
   These changes are diagnostic of pregnancy.
   a. This is not considered a categorical change of pregnancy.
   b. These symptoms suggest but do not confirm pregnancy.
   c. These changes strongly suggest pregnancy, but are not diagnostic.
   Comprehensive/Physiologic/Assessment

9. **Correct response: b**
   Nausea is a presumptive sign of pregnancy.
   a, c, and d. Goodall's sign, skin changes, and positive pregnancy test are all probable signs of pregnancy.
   Knowledge/Physiologic/Assessment

10. *Correct response: d*

The second trimester normally is a relatively tranquil time; the woman typically feels only minor discomfort and has physically adjusted to the pregnancy. Excitement about the pregnancy typically develops once quickening has occurred.

a and b. These may occur; however, they are not major factors in maternal well-being.

c. Acceptance of the neonate does not occur until after birth.

Knowledge/Psychosocial/Assessment

Childbirth Education

I. Overview

A. Essential concepts

1. The term natural childbirth initially described for many people a particular childbirth approach (e.g., delivery without analgesia or anesthesia). To those who developed the approach, however, it primarily meant being prepared for childbirth.

2. Prepared childbirth more accurately describes the prenatal education education training to deal with the discomforts of labor and delivery.

3. More and more families in all socioeconomic groups are participating in prepared childbirth classes.

4. In order to act as a resource for parents, the nurse needs to have factual information about the range of techniques taught in the various prepared childbirth approaches.

5. Regardless of approach, all types of childbirth classes commonly provide information about prenatal care and planning for birth,

fetal growth and development, preparation for labor and delivery, and postpartum care of mother and infant.

6. Inclusion of fathers in the birthing process has become an increasingly important aspect of prepared childbirth.

7. Prepared childbirth has become a standard part of prenatal care in the United States, with a number of maternity centers sponsoring classes for their clients.

8. Components of childbirth preparation include:
    a. Education, focusing on prenatal care, nutrition, infant care and feeding, labor and delivery, cesarean birth, and postpartum care
    b. Training, involving practicing exercises and breathing techniques

9. Because individuals vary in their response to stress and because the character of individual labor varies, the judicious use of pain medication along with breathing and relaxation may enhance the woman's ability to use relaxation techniques successfully.

10. The relatively uneventful second trimester offers a good opportunity for learning about childbirth and parenting.

11. Goals of prepared childbirth include:
    a. Provide parents with knowledge and skills necessary to cope with the stresses of pregnancy, labor, and birth.
    b. Prepare parents to be knowledgeable health care consumers.
    c. Assist parents in achieving a positive, safe, and rewarding labor and birth experience.

B. **Parental decisions**
    1. Some childbearing couples select their primary birthing attendant (e.g., obstetrician) and allow the attendant to make decisions on their behalf. Other couples decide what they want in the childbearing experience and choose their primary birthing attendant accordingly.
    2. Decisions to be made by the childbearing couple include:
        a. Determining where they prefer to deliver the infant (e.g., hospital with traditional maternity center or birthing center, community agency, private hospital, freestanding birthing center, home)
        b. Selecting birthing attendant (e.g., obstetrician, pediatrician, family practice physician, midwife)
        c. Selecting a preferred birthing approach and devising a birth plan
    3. Couples need to understand how birth plans can be modified to meet the specific demands and changes of their birth experience.

C. **Effectiveness of prepared childbirth**
    1. The stress reduction and relaxation techniques learned help the woman cope more effectively with the stress of labor.

2. Unsupported claims include supporting parent–infant bonding, improving the spouses' relationship, and facilitating painless labor.
3. Prepared childbirth may enhance neonatal health if it eliminates or minimizes the use of analgesics and anesthetics during labor and delivery.

II. Prenatal and postpartum teaching
A. Prenatal education programs
1. These programs vary widely in length, goals, and content.
2. First trimester classes commonly focus on such issues as early physiologic changes, fetal development, sexuality during pregnancy, and nutrition; some early classes may include prepregnant couples.
3. Second and third trimester classes may focus on preparation for birth, parenting, and infant care.

B. Postpartum education programs
1. With the emergence of shorter hospital stays, classes following delivery are increasingly being offered through hospitals, clinics, private agencies, and health professionals in private practice.
2. Although these programs vary widely in length, goals, and content, they all provide support for parents.
3. These programs often are extensions of the prenatal classes and deal with issues as they emerge from parents' concerns (e.g., mother's body image concerns, fertility and infertility, parenting).

C. Content of childbirth education classes
1. Prenatal care and planning
   a. Nutrition, exercise, rest
   b. Parental discomforts and self-care measures
   c. Making a birth plan
   d. Choosing a birth setting, primary care provider, and birth approach
   e. Recognition of danger signs and symptoms
2. Fetal development
   a. Maternal drug and medication use
   b. Maternal nutrition
   c. Environmental hazards
   d. Developmental milestones
3. Preparation for labor and delivery
   a. Muscle toning exercises
   b. Breathing techniques
   c. Relaxation exercises
   d. Analgesia and anesthesia
   f. Preparation for possible cesarean delivery
4. Postpartum care

      a.   Self-care
      b.   Neonatal care
      c.   Feeding methods
      d.   Maternal nutrition, exercise, and rest needs
      e.   Recognition of danger signs and symptoms

D. **Teaching methods**
  1.   Individual teaching and counseling
  2.   Groups and classes structured as informational classes, counseling groups, or discussion groups

E. **Approaches to childbirth education**
  1.   Grantly Dick-Read suggests that education decreases fear, tension, and pain, and teaches exercises to improve muscle tone and increase relaxation and stresses slow breathing, muscle relaxation, and pushing techniques.
  2.   The Lamaze or psychoprophylactic method combines relaxation, concentration, focusing, and complex breathing patterns to reduce perception of pain through a conditioned response to labor contractions.
  3.   The Bradley techniques focus on slow breathing and deep relaxation for labor and reduced responsiveness to external stimuli and the role for the male partner as coach; it is basically Dick-Read's approach with the addition of a labor coach.
  4.   The Wright or "new childbirth" method involves less active breathing than in the Lamaze method, with breathing patterns increasing in complexity as labor progresses.
  5.   The Kitzinger method uses sensory memory as an aid to understanding and working with the body in preparation for childbirth.
  6.   Yoga teaches relaxation, concentration, and "complete breathing" (combination of chest and abdominal breathing).
  7.   Hypnosis may be of benefit for some patients.
  8.   Contemporary childbirth education methods tend to be eclectic, combining features of many approaches, particularly Dick-Read, Lamaze, and Bradley.

F. **Sibling preparation classes**
  1.   Purposes include preparing children for what to expect when they visit mother and new baby in the hospital, reducing the problems associated with separation when mother goes to the hospital, and facilitating the parents' preparation of children for the introduction of the new baby in the home.
  2.   There are a few programs that prepare children for attendance at birth; a sibling-support person is usually expected to accompany the child to reduce distraction of mother during labor.

G. **Grandparent preparation classes**
  1.   Classes frequently offered in maternity centers that encourage

grandparent visits, including holding the newborn, with extended visiting hours

    2. Purposes include increasing grandparents' awareness of changes that have occurred in childbearing and childrearing and increasing grandparents' awareness of their own feelings.

    3. Some grandparents are an integral part of the birthing experience and as such also need information about being a "coach."

    4. The need for knowledgeable extended family support systems becomes increasingly important with shorter hospital stays.

H. Breast-feeding programs

    1. Content includes preparation of breasts, techniques for breast-feeding, and advantages vs. disadvantages

    2. Offered by hospitals, birthing centers, clinics, individuals, and the LaLeche League

    3. Fathers are being included more frequently, because these provide opportunity for expression of their feelings—both positive and negative—about breast-feeding.

III. Implications for nursing

A. Assessment

    1. Determine the woman's or couple's expectations about the class and about childbirth.

    2. Evaluate knowledge of:

        a. Anatomy and physiology of pregnancy

        b. Fetal development

        c. What to expect during prenatal visits

        d. Preparation for labor and delivery

        e. Infant care

        f. Self-care

B. Nursing diagnoses

    1. Anxiety

    2. Fear

    3. Knowledge Deficit

    4. Noncompliance

    5. Powerlessness

C. Planning and implementation

    1. Use standard adult-learning principles in childbirth education.

    2. After assessing individual or group needs, provide instruction as needed on such topics as:

        a. Minor discomforts and their alleviation

        b. Fetal growth and development

        c. Nutritional needs during pregnancy and lactation

        d. Newborn care, such as sleeping and waking patterns, infant safety, bathing and feeding techniques, cord care, pros and cons of circumcision

        e. Prenatal assessment and diagnostic testing of fetal status

(e.g., complete blood profile, urinalysis, ultrasonography routinely, with at-risk patients possibly undergoing maternal–fetal activity assessment, estriol determinations, nonstress test, contraction stress test, or amniocentesis)

f. Danger signs and symptoms (e.g., spotting, headaches, edema, unusual pain, increased temperature, painful urination, signs of preterm labor)

g. Preparation for labor and delivery (e.g., signs and symptoms of true labor, when to go to the hospital or call the physician or midwife, plans for getting to the hospital with alternate options, what to expect during admission process, what to expect of medical and nursing care, fetal monitoring techniques and purpose, breathing techniques during labor, relaxation techniques in between contractions, analgesia during labor and delivery, hydration during labor)

h. Preparation for infant feeding, including advantages and disadvantages of breast-feeding and bottle-feeding:

   (1) Bottle feeding: advantages (e.g., prepared to be as much like breast milk as possible, can tell how much the baby is taking, father can enhance bonding during feeding, easier to satisfy large babies), disadvantages (e.g., some babies become colicky, decreased transfer of immune bodies from mother); preparation for (e.g., powder and liquid preparation chance of error in preparation, less expensive, prepared formulas that need refrigeration must be rewarmed, prepared formulas may be quite expensive)

   (2) Breast-feeding: advantages (e.g., considered to be the best food for neonate, involution occurs more rapidly, readily available, no preparation needed, no cost) disadvantages (e.g., father cannot feed, takes 3 weeks to be fully established, which may be frustrating for a large baby); preparation for (e.g., providing literature, demonstrating nipple preparation, facilitating psychological preparation for the demands of breast-feeding)

i. Preparation for analgesia and anesthesia during labor and delivery, including advantages and disadvantages of available options: natural childbirth, regional anesthesia, systemic medications, inhalation anesthesia, general anesthesia

j. Sibling preparation for birth, including:

   (1) Involvement of children during antepartal period and labor and delivery (e.g., listening to fetal

heart tones, feeling the baby move and kick, naming the baby, doll play)
    (2) Intrapartal visitation, advantages and disadvantages, preparation for holding the newborn
    (3) Postpartum sibling visits, early discharge of mother, sibling involvement in helping mother
    (4) Expecting and coping with sibling rivalry (e.g., providing extra attention, considering arriving home without baby to give siblings undivided attention before introducing newborn to the home)
  k. Grandparent preparation for birth, including:
    (1) Community support classes
    (2) Discussions on how to provide help without "smothering" parents (e.g., when to babysit)
    (3) Preparation for involvement during labor and delivery
  l. Preparation for possible cesarean birth, including indications, advantages and disadvantages, risks, partner's involvement, anesthesia

3. Integrate the father into preparation for childbirth by providing such information as:
  a. How to coach the mother during labor and delivery
  b. The importance of helping spouse keep antenatal appointments
  c. The significance of fetal heart tones (FHTs) and the sonogram; encouraging him to listen to FHTs and view the sonogram
  d. How he can participate in preparing the home environment for the new baby
  e. Preparing siblings for the new infant

D. Evaluation
1. The expectant parents verbalize satisfaction with plans for delivery and choice of primary caregiver.
2. The parents demonstrate understanding of the assessments and diagnostic tests done during pregnancy.
3. The father verbalizes understanding of his role in the childbirth process.
4. The couple verbalizes understanding of the major concepts and content of childbirth education classes.
5. The parents are able to discuss with the primary caregiver the options for analgesia and anesthesia.
6. The parents state the circumstances that may necessitate a cesarean birth.
7. The parents verbalize danger signs and the need to report them promptly.

8. The parents explore various feeding methods.

9. The mother verbalizes important aspects of infant care and self-care in the postpartum period.

Bibliography

Danforth, D. N. (Ed.) (1986). *Obstetrics and gynecology* (5th ed.). Philadelphia: J. B. Lippincott.

Jensen, M. D., & Bobak, I. M. (1985). *Maternity and gynecologic care: The nurse and family* (3rd ed.). St. Louis: C. V. Mosby.

May, K. A., & Mahlmeister, L. R. (1990). *Comprehensive maternity nursing: Nursing process and the childbearing family* (2nd ed.). Philadelphia: J. B. Lippincott.

Olds, S. (1984). *Maternity-newborn nursing*. Menlo Park, CA: Addison-Wesley.

Reeder, S. J., & Martin, L. L. (1987). *Maternity nursing: Family, newborn, and women's health care* (16th ed.). Philadelphia: J. B. Lippincott.

STUDY QUESTIONS

1. Preparation for childbirth education often includes postpartum physiological and psychological adjustment of the mother, with little emphasis on the baby. Which of the following is the best reason for covering this content during the prenatal period?
   a. With early discharge, the nurse cannot teach both mother and baby care during postpartum.
   b. Mothers are more ready to learn infant care after the baby is born, but can learn some postpartum self-care before delivery.
   c. Mothers need to learn postpartum self-care and neonatal care after delivery.
   d. Mothers are more interested in learning about labor and delivery than postpartum changes.

2. A patient asks the nurse, "How will I know when I'm in true labor?" Which of the following would be the nurse's best response?
   a. "The mucous plug will be released."
   b. "Contractions will occur at irregular intervals."
   c. "Contractions will increase in intensity and duration."
   d. "You'll feel contractions in the lower abdomen."

3. The best definition of prepared childbirth is which of the following?
   a. preparation of the room, layette, and equipment ready for the birth
   b. classes about pregnancy and parenting
   c. family-centered counseling that prepares family members for the crisis of birth
   d. prenatal education to deal with the discomfort of labor and delivery

4. Which of the following would the nurse providing childbirth preparation *not* encourage parents to finalize?
   a. location of delivery (e.g., hospital, birthing center, home)
   b. birthing attendant (e.g., obstetrician, midwife)
   c. type of delivery (e.g., vaginal, cesarean section)
   d. birth plan

5. During childbirth preparation classes, the nurse always has the learners and their coaches practice what has been demonstrated. Which of the following principles is the basis for this action?
   a. Learning is directly influenced by the physical and social environment.
   b. Learners are motivated by teacher acceptance.
   c. Learners ultimately learn what they desire to learn.
   d. Learning is enhanced when learning provides opportunity for application.

6. A primary difference between the Dick-Read and Bradley methods of childbirth preparation is which of the following?
   a. Dick-Read suggested hypnosis, whereas Bradley did not.
   b. Bradley added the idea of the coach to Dick-Read's approach.
   c. Bradley added a more focused yoga concentration aspect.
   d. Dick-Read placed more emphasis on "mind prevention."

7. Mary Ann Markey has enrolled her 9-year-old daughter in a sibling preparation class. Which of the following is *not* usually a major focus of these classes?
   a. what to expect when they visit their mother and new baby in the hospital
   b. dealing with the separation caused by the mother's hospitalization
   c. how it feels to have a new baby sister or brother in the home
   d. how to provide basic child care and safe babysitting

8. When conducting a "preparation for infant feeding" unit in a childbirth education series, which of the following would be *incorrect* to teach as an advantage of bottle feeding?
   a. Involution occurs more rapidly be-

cause hormones can more readily regain balance.
b. The father can more readily bond
with infant through feeding.
c. The amount of intake of milk is more
readily determined.
d. It may be easier to satisfy large babies.

ANSWER KEY

1. *Correct response: b*
   Pregnant women tend to be narcissistic and self-focused about labor, delivery, and postpartum recovery prenatally and are more interested in infant care once the baby arrives.
   a, c, and d. Both self-care and baby care should be dealt with during the postpartum period, despite the woman's inattention and early discharge.
   Application/Health promotion/Planning

2. *Correct response: c*
   Increased intensity and duration of contractions is the most accurate symptom of labor.
   a. The mucous plug may or may not be released.
   b. Contractions occur at regular intervals.
   d. Contractions start in the back and sweep around to the front.
   Application/Physiologic/Implementation

3. *Correct response: d*
   Prepared childbirth involves prenatal education to help the mother and partner understand and deal with labor and delivery.
   a, b, and c. These may be included in prenatal education discussions, but are not specific to prepared childbirth.
   Comprehensive/Health promotion/Planning

4. *Correct response: c*
   Although a couple may prefer a certain type of delivery, they should understand that the final choice regarding delivery will be based on maternal and fetal safety.
   a, b, and d. A couple can plan on the location of delivery, choose a birthing attendant, and make a birth plan while they await onset of labor.
   Application/Safe care/Implementation

5. *Correct response: d*
   The most effective learning occurs when it provides opportunities for application.
   a, b, and c. Although these are important principles, they are not directly related to learner involvement in practicing learned skills.
   Application/Health promotion/Implementation

6. *Correct response: b*
   Dick-Read's and Bradley's approaches both involve slow breathing and muscle relaxation, but Bradley introduced the coach.
   a, c, and d. These responses don't reflect the differences between the Dick-Read and Bradley approaches.
   Knowledge/Health promotion/Implementation

7. *Correct response: d*
   Although classes may discuss how to treat and handle the baby, child care and babysitting are not usually major aspects of preparing siblings for the pending birth.
   a, b, and c. These are all common aspects of sibling preparation.
   Comprehensive/Health promotion/Planning

8. *Correct response: a*
   Involution occurs more readily with breast-feeding, not bottle feeding.
   b, c, and d. These responses are all correct information about bottle feeding.
   Application/Health promotion/Implementation

Antepartal Care

8

I. Overview

A. **Essential concepts**

1. Antepartal care refers to the medical and nursing care given to the pregnant woman between conception and the onset of labor.

2. Consideration is given to the physical, emotional, and social needs of the woman, the unborn child, her partner, and other family members.

3. Pregnancy is viewed as a normal physiologic process, not a disease process; nevertheless, at no other time in life does a healthy woman need such intense, regular care as during pregnancy.

4. With the advent of highly sophisticated instrumentation and monitoring, the nurse must be particularly alert that these techniques are used to augment practice and should never replace the therapeutic process.
5. The value of prenatal care in terms of maternal–fetal outcome is well documented.
6. However, prenatal care—even of the highest quality—does not guarantee a positive outcome.
7. The process of data gathering and analysis is ongoing; the nurse cannot expect to cover all areas during the initial antepartal visit, and so should focus on trimester-specific issues.

B. Goals of antepartal care
1. Increase the expectant mother's and family's knowledge of pregnancy and the actions they can take to facilitate a positive birth outcome.
2. Assist all family members to experience pregnancy in a positive way.
3. Promote successful integration of the new baby into the family.

C. Factors affecting the antepartal experience
1. Previous experience with pregnancy
2. Cultural and personal expectations
3. Prepregnant health and biophysical preparedness for childbearing
4. Motivation for childbearing
5. Socioeconomic status
6. Mother's age and partnered vs. unpartnered status
7. Accessibility of prenatal care

D. Nursing responsibilities
1. Perform trimester-specific physiologic and psychosocial assessment and facilitate follow-up care as needed.
2. Provide education and counseling for the pregnant woman and her family.
3. Make appropriate referrals for additional services as needed.

II. Essentials of antepartal assessment
A. Health history
1. Current pregnancy: first day of last menstrual period, cramping or bleeding, results of pregnancy test, discomfort (e.g., nausea, vomiting, headache, frequency, fatigue)
2. History of previous pregnancies: gravida, para, number of abortions, number of living children, prenatal education
3. Gynecologic history: previous infections; previous surgery; age of menarche and menstrual cycle; sexual, menstrual, and contraception history
4. Current medical history: weight, blood type and Rh, medications presently taking (prescription and over-the-counter), habits (smoking, alcohol, caffeine, drugs), allergies, potential terato-

genic effects on this pregnancy (infections, medications, radiographs, etc, toxins in home or workplace), medical conditions (diabetes, hypertension, cardiovascular, renal, congenital), immunizations

5. Past medical history: childhood diseases, medical diseases and treatment, history of sexually transmitted diseases, past surgeries, bleeding disorders or past blood transfusions, emotional problems, accidents

6. Family medical history: medical disorders (e.g., cancer, heart disease, diabetes), multiple births, genetic or congenital disorders, cesarean births

7. Occupational history: type of work and health hazards

8. History of father of baby: age, health problems, habits, blood type and Rh, genetic or congenital disorders, occupation, attitude toward pregnancy

9. Personal information: race, cultural, and religious patterns; exercise; housing and living conditions; income; support system; use of health care system; work

B. Assessment of risk factors

1. Early identification of factors that place mother and baby at risk provides opportunity for interventions to mitigate the associated dangers.

2. Risk factors that could have a negative effect on the pregnancy may be characterized as demographic, obstetric, medical, and miscellaneous (Table 8–1).

C. Diagnostic tests and procedures

1. During the initial assessment of physical status, which typically occurs during the first prenatal visits, baseline data are obtained, providing a measure against which subsequent data are evaluated.

2. Laboratory tests include:
   a. Urine tests: protein, glucose, ketones, bilirubin, blood, white blood cells, bacteria
   b. Blood tests: hemoglobin and hematocrit, blood type, Rh, and antibody titer; rubella screen, serology, hemoglobin electrophoresis, hepatitis B, human immunodeficiency virus (HIV) testing
   c. Diabetes screen: usually done at 24 to 28 weeks because of hormonal effects that block insulin usage
   d. Cultures: Pap, gonorrhea, vaginal smear

III. Evaluation of fetal well-being

A. Essential concepts

1. Monitoring of maternal weight gain, uterine growth, fetal activity, and fetal heart rate (FHR) is usually done at each prenatal visit.

2. In approximately 20% of pregnancies, further assessment of fetal well-being is indicated.

TABLE 8-1.
Perinatal Risk Assessment

AREAS TO BE ASSESSED	CONDITIONS ASSOCIATED WITH INCREASED RISK

Antepartal Course

General prenatal information — Lack of prenatal care
Weight gain $\leq$ 15 lb or $\geq$ 35 lb

Maternal health — Medical conditions:
 Diabetes
  Insulin-dependent*
 Heart disease
Habits:
 Smoking
 Substance abuse
Infections during prengancy:
 Rubella
 Venereal disease
Complications of pregnancy:
 Pregnancy-induced hypertension
 3rd-trimester bleeding*
 Rh sensitization
  Severe*
 Multiple fetuses*

Results of antepartal tests — Estriol levels: $\downarrow$ or no $\uparrow$ after 36 wk
Ultrasound: growth retardation $\geq$ 2 wk
Amniocentesis:
 Bilirubin or meconium present
 L/S ratio $<$ 2:1
Nonstress test: nonreactive
Stress test: positive

Intrapartum Course

Length of pregnancy — $\leq$ 37 week; $\geq$ 42 wk; * $<$ 34 wk
Duration and character of labor — *Prolonged 1st or 2nd stage
Precipitous labor or delivery
PROM $>$ 24 h
Difficult labor
Cephalopelvic disproportion

Maternal conditions — Preexisting problems (see antepartal course)
Progressive hypotension
Progressive hypertension
Excessive bleeding*
Signs of Infection
 Severe*

Fetal presentation and position — Breech*
Transverse lie*

Events indicating possible fetal distress — Fetal monitoring
 Persistent late decelerations*
 Severe variable decelerations*
 Heart Rate $<$ 120 or $>$ 160 for $>$ 30 min
 Poor beat-to-beat variability*
Scalp pH $\leq$ 7.25*
Meconium-stained fluid*
Prolapsed cord*

(continued)

TABLE 8-1.
Perinatal Risk Assessment (Continued)

AREAS TO BE ASSESSED	CONDITIONS ASSOCIATED WITH INCREASED RISK
Analgesia	Large or repeated doses of analgesia
	IM analgesia witin 1 h of delivery
	IV analgesia within $\frac{1}{2}$ h of delivery
Anesthesia	General anesthesia
	Conduction anesthesia with maternal hypotension
Method of Delivery	Cesarean delivery*
	Mid forceps or high forceps delivery*
	Failed vacuum extraction

* *Conditions ususally requiring presence at delivery of someone skilled in resuscitation.*

3. First-trimester fetal assessments typically include auscultation of FHR and ultrasonography.
4. Second-trimester assessments typically include measurements of fundal height, FHR, fetal movement (quickening), and ultrasonography.
5. Aspects of third-trimester assessment include monitoring fetal movement and ultrasonography.

B. FHR
1. FHR usually is auscultated at the midline suprapubic region with a Doptone (ultrasound stethoscope) at 10 to 12 weeks' gestation.
2. FHR can be auscultated with a fetoscope at about 20 weeks' gestation.
3. A FHR of 120 to 160 beats per minute can be distinguished from the slower maternal rate by simultaneously palpating the mother's pulse.
4. FHR is determined at each visit.
5. A regular heart beat is normal; irregularity is abnormal.
6. The heart beat will be muffled when the mother's abdominal wall is thick, if she is obese, or if there is a large amount of amniotic fluid.
7. Fundic souffle, caused by the rushing of blood through the umbilical arteries, is synchronous with the FHR; uterine souffle, sound of blood passing through the uterine blood vessels, is synchronous with the maternal pulse.
8. Failure to hear FHR may result from inexperience with fetoscope, defective fetoscope or a noisy environment, early pregnancy and small-for-gestational-age fetus, fetal death, obesity, hydramnios, loud placental souffle obscuring the FHR, and posterior position of the fetus.

C. Ultrasonography (sonograms)
1. Serial sonograms provide much useful information in assessing fetal growth and well-being.

2. Ultrasonography provides different information during different trimesters:
   a. First trimester
      (1) Assessment of gestational age
      (2) Evaluation for congenital anomalies
      (3) Diagnostic evaluation of vaginal bleeding
      (4) Confirmation of suspected multiple gestation
      (5) Evaluation of fetal growth
      (6) Adjunct to prenatal testing (amniocentesis, chorionic villus sampling)
      (7) Diagnostic evaluation of pelvic mass
   b. Second trimester
      (1) Assessment of gestational age
      (2) Evaluation of congenital anomalies (e.g., hydrocephaly)
      (3) Assessment of fetal growth
      (4) Guidance of procedures, such as amniocentesis and fetoscopy
      (5) Assessment of placental location
      (6) Diagnosis of multiple gestation
   c. Third trimester
      (1) Determination of fetal position
      (2) Estimation of fetal size
3. Second-trimester sonogram is recommended as a baseline for all pregnancies considered to be at risk for complications.
4. A full bladder may improve ultrasonic resolution before 20 weeks' gestation, and mothers may be instructed to drink a quart or more of fluids 1 to 2 hours before the procedure during the first trimester.
5. When used as an adjunct to prenatal diagnoses, visualization of the baby may contribute to the difficulty of pregnancy termination decisions.
6. It is possible to visualize head, extremities, moving heart valves and, frequently, to determine the sex of the fetus. The parental desire to know the sex of the child should be ascertained before providing this information.

D. Measurement of fundal height
1. Begin during the second trimester when the fundus is palpable until the end of pregnancy
2. McDonald's measurement: using a nonstretching but flexible measuring tape, place the zero point on the superior border of the symphysis pubis and stretch the tape across the abdomen at the midline to the top of the fundus.
3. After 20 to 22 weeks, the fundal height in centimeters normally approximates the gestational age in weeks

4. Possible causes of greater-than-expected fundal height include multiple gestation, polyhydramnios, and fetal macrosomia
5. Possible causes for less-than-expected fundal height include abnormal fetal presentation, fetal growth retardation, congenital anomalies, and oligohydramnios

E. Fetal movement or quickening
1. In primigravidas, quickening normally is detected between 18 and 20 weeks' gestation.
2. In secundigravidas and multigravidas, this may occur as early as 16 weeks.
3. Quickening is typically described as a light fluttering feeling; it may be mistaken for flatus.

F. Electronic fetal heart monitoring (EFHM)
1. EFHM is used during the antepartal period to evaluate a high-risk fetus.
2. It demonstrates fetal heart response to spontaneous or induced uterine contractions.
3. Contractions stress the fetus by decreasing uterine perfusion. In a fetus already compromised by disease, cord compression, or other factors, contractions may alter heart rate, detectable on EFHM.
4. Common EFHM methods include the nonstress test and the contraction stress test.
5. Nonstress test (NST)
   a. This is the least invasive test of fetal well-being, involving the use of an electronic fetal monitor. The baseline FHR and the presence of periodic patterns are identified and correlated to contractions observed on the uterine activity tracing.
   b. Adequate perfusion is necessary to maintain fetal central nervous system integrity and reflex responses.
   c. A healthy fetus responds to fetal movement with an accelerated heart rate; in this case, the test is said to be negative or reactive.
   d. Among the various assessment protocols, the most common involves two FHR accelerations within a 10-minute period, with each accleration increasing heart rate by at least 15 beats per minute and lasting at least 15 seconds.
   e. The fetus typically is monitored for at least 40 minutes (to account for a normal sleep period), then the entire tracing is evaluated.
   f. An abnormal or nonreactive NST requires further evaluation that same day.
   g. Even with a reactive NST, follow-up is indicated if FHR falls outside the range of 120 to 160 beats per minute or if decelerations (early, late, or variable) are detected.

7. Contraction stress test
   a. Perfusion through the spinal arteries of the uterus is decreased during contractions; the fetus with limited reserve responds to the stress of contractions with late decelerations, while the healthy fetus displays a normal pattern with no decelerations.
   b. During fetal testing, contractions may occur spontaneously; most often, however, stimulation will be necessary. This is done either by breast stimulation (e.g., nipple rolling, application of moist hot pads) to trigger prolactin release or by low-dose oxytocin infusion (oxytocin challenge test [OCT]).
   c. Three contractions within 10 minutes—ideally, lasting 40 to 60 seconds each—must be evaluated to assess fetal response to stress.
   d. During an OCT, the nurse must keep in mind that oxytocin may precipitate labor.

G. **Other procedures to evaluate fetal well-being**
   1. Amniocentesis can determine fetal maturity and detect certain birth defects (e.g., Down's syndrome, spina bifida), hemolytic disease of the newborn, and gender and chromosomal abnormalities.
   2. Chorionic villus biopsy is done early in pregnancy to detect fetal abnormalities.
   3. Other routine tests include maternal urine and serum assays.
   4. Fetoscopy involves direct fetal visualization through a telescope introduced through the abdominal and uterine walls.
   5. Amnioscopy (transcervical fetal visualization) and radiographs are less commonly done.

IV. **Nursing management during the normal anterpartal period**
   A. **Initial assessment**
      1. Vital signs, height, and weight (current and prepregnant)
      2. Systematic, thorough physical examination, including pelvic examination
      3. Determination of estimated date of delivery (EDD) or estimated date of confinement
         a. Average length of pregnancy is 280 days (40 weeks, 10 lunar months, or 9 calendar months), as calculated from the first day of the last menstrual period (LMP)
         b. Dating pregnancy when LMP is known by Nagele's rule: take the first day of LMP, subtract 7 days, and then add 3 months to arrive at the EDD
         c. Dating pregnancy when LMP is unknown:
            (1) Uterine size is reported in terms of weeks of gestation at the first prenatal visit.
            (2) Presence of the uterus in the abdomen (fundal height) indicates at least 12 weeks' gestation.

(3) Presence of the uterus in the pelvis (fundal height) indicates less than 12 weeks' gestation.

(4) Quickening (fetal movement felt by the mother) indicates about 20 weeks' gestation in primigravidas; less in multigravidas.

(5) Fetal heart tones can be detected at 10 to 12 weeks' gestation with Doppler and at 16 to 20 weeks with a fetoscope.

(6) Ultrasound can detect pregnancy 5 to 6 weeks after last menstrual period.

4. Assessment of pelvic size for adequacy (See Chapter 2 for discussion of pelvic measurements.):

   a. Measurement of the dimensions and proportion of the bony pelvis

   b. Obtained during bimanual portion of the pelvic examination by moving the fingers over the landmarks of the bony pelvis and estimating their size

   c. May be delayed until later in pregnancy when the procedure may be more comfortable for the mother, because it is not crucial to determine pelvic adequacy this early in pregnancy

5. Inspection and palpation of breasts for normal changes of pregnancy and questionable changes

   a. Normal changes associated with pregnancy (e.g., increased size, tenderness, darkening and enlargement of areola, erection of nipples and leaking of colostrum late in first trimester, appearance of venous pattern and striae formation)

   b. Questionable changes (e.g., recent lumps or masses that feel hard or fixed, dimpling, redness, edema, ulceration, nipple retraction or elevation)

6. Psychosocial assessment during initial visit(s) may include:

   a. Determining expectations for pregnancy, emotional and financial impact on family, partner's attitude toward pregnancy (e.g., excitement or apprehension)

   b. Whether or not the pregnancy was planned

   c. Educational needs and resources

   d. Support systems

   e. Religious beliefs and cultural practices related to childbirth and parenting

   f. Family functioning, living situation, sexual activity

   g. Preparation for parenthood; preparation for childbirth

B. Subsequent prenatal visit assessments

1. Frequency of prenatal visits: every 4 weeks for the first 28 weeks; every 2 weeks to 36 weeks; then weekly until delivery

2. Physical assessment with each prenatal visit includes the following:

      a.   Data concerning course of pregnancy (e.g., common discomforts and how alleviated)

      b.   Maternal vital signs: temperature, pulse, respiration, and blood pressure

      c.   Weight gain (distribution per trimester)

      d.   Presence of edema

      e.   Uterine size (ballottement and engagement)

      f.   FHR

      g.   Urine for protein and glucose

      h.   Danger signals: vaginal bleeding, blurred vision, leaking of amniotic fluid, rapid weight gain, elevated blood pressure

      i.   After 38 weeks, signs of impending labor: lightening, engagement, cervical status

  3. Laboratory tests include:

      a.   Urine dipstick for glucose, protein, ketones each visit

      b.   Complete blood count or Hgb, Hct each trimester

      c.   Rh antibody screen at 24 to 28 weeks if negative or previous sensitization

      d.   Sexually transmitted disease (STD) tests repeated if indicated

      e.   Blood glucose screen at 24 to 28 weeks

  4. Also evaluate educational needs relative to sexual activity, preparation for parenting, preparation for childbirth, knowledge of signs of labor.

  5. Assess psychologic and emotional status; allow the patient or couple time to ask questions and express concerns.

  6. Perform a nutritional assessment, including:

      a.   Review of dietary intake of iron, iron supplements

      b.   24-hour diet recall

      c.   Comparison of prepregnancy weight to weight gained during pregnancy (over the course of the pregnancy, a total weight gain of 25 to 30 lb is recommended)

      d.   Pattern of weight gain (normal is 1.5 lb in the first 10 weeks; 9.0 lb at 20 weeks; 19 lb by 30 weeks; and 27.5 lb by 40 weeks)

      e.   Nondietary factors affecting weight gain (e.g., increased blood pressure and excess fluid retention)

  C. **Assessment of common minor discomforts of pregnancy**

    1. First trimester

      a.   Nausea and vomiting (morning sickness): generally occurs after first missed menstrual period and subsides by the fourth month of pregnancy; is due to change in hormone levels

      b.   Nasal stuffiness and epistaxis: due to nasal edema from elevated estrogen levels

      c.   Urinary frequency: caused by pressure of growing uterus on bladder; seen in first trimester and again in the later part of the third trimester

    d.   Breast tenderness: occurs early in pregnancy and continues throughout due to hormonal change

    e.   Ptyalism: excessive salvation

    f.   Leukorrhea: increased vaginal discharge

    g.   Headaches: due to emotional tension, eye strains, vascular engorgement, and congestion of sinuses from hormonal stimulation

    h.   Stuffy nose: congestion due to hormone stimulation

2.   Second and third trimesters

    a.   Heartburn due to regurgitation of acidic gastric contents into the esophagus; may be associated with tension and vomiting in the third trimester

    b.   Ankle edema due to decreased venous return in the lower extremities

    c.   Varicose veins due to poor circulation and weakened vessel walls

    d.   Hemorrhoids due to pressure of the gravid uterus on the spine, which interferes with venous circulation

    e.   Constipation due to decreased peristalsis of the bowel and displacement of intestines from a gravid uterus, insufficient fluid intake, or use of iron supplements

    f.   Backache resulting from altered posture due to increased curvature of the lumbosacral vertebrae from the enlarging uterus

    g.   Leg cramps from spasms of the gastrocnemius muscle

    h.   Faintness due to changes in blood volume and postural hypotension

    i.   Shortness of breath due to pressure exerted on the diaphragm by an enlarging uterus

    j.   Difficulty sleeping due to an enlarged uterus

    k.   Round ligament pain due to stretching and hypertrophy of the ligaments

D.   **Nursing diagnoses**

    1.   Anxiety

    2.   Body Image Disturbance

    3.   Altered Bowel Elimination

    4.   Ineffective Family Coping: High Risk for Growth

    5.   Fear

    6.   Health-seeking Behaviors

    7.   Knowledge Deficit

    8.   Altered Nutrition: Less than Body Requirements

    9.   Altered Nutrition: More than Body Requirements

    10.   Altered Role Performance

    11.   Self-concept Disturbance

12. Altered Patterns of Sexuality
13. Sexual Dysfunction

E. Planning and implementation: first trimester

1. Maintain good nutritional status. Stress well-balanced meals; review basic four food groups, vitamin and mineral supplementation.
2. Increase fluid intake to prevent urinary tract infection and improve kidney function.
3. Intervene to relieve common discomforts:
    a. Nausea: instruct to eat small, dry, bland meals, taking fluids between meals; encourage a snack of dry crackers before arising.
    b. Tiredness: instruct to rest whenever possible, get at least 8 hours of sleep each night, and elevate legs when sitting.
    c. Nasal stuffiness: instruct to use a cool air vaporizer or humidifier, maintain increased fluid intake, place moist towel on sinuses, massage sinuses.
    d. Urinary frequency: encourage to void when urge felt and decrease fluid intake in evening.
    e. Breast tenderness: instruct in wearing of a supportive brassiere.
    e. Ptyalism: encourage use of mouthwash, chewing gum, or sucking on hard candy.
    f. Leukorrhea: instruct to bathe daily; avoid douching, and wear nylon undergarments and panty hose.
    g. Headaches: instruct to get enough sleep and rest; eat regular meals; drink fluids; apply cool washcloth to head and back of neck; massage neck, shoulders, face, scalp, forehead; take warm bath; relax and meditate.
4. Discuss sexual concerns with the patient and partner as appropriate; cover reasons for altered libido (increased or decreased).

F. Planning and implementation: second and third trimesters

1. Continue to address nutritional needs; assess for normal weight gain.
2. Intervene for common discomforts:
    a. Heartburn: encourage to eat small frequent meals and avoid overeating, and spicy, fatty, and fried foods.
    b. Ankle edema: elevate legs when resting and caution against wearing tight garters on legs.
    c. Varicose veins: instruct to elevate legs, wear supportive hose, and avoid garters, crossing legs, or standing for long periods of time.
    d. Hemorrhoids: encourage regulation of bowel habit with use of stool softener, use of cold packs or sitz baths, glycerine suppositories, and gentle reinsertion of hemorrhoid with lubricated fingers, diet with adequate roughage.

    e. Constipation: discuss the importance of adequate dietary fiber intake, increased fluid intake, and exercise; allow use of milk of magnesia, but avoid strong laxatives.

    f. Backache: encourage to maintain good posture and to do the pelvic tilt exercise; encourage not to stand or sit for long periods of time and to distribute body weight by altering stance.

    g. Leg cramps: increase calcium and decrease phosphorous intake, evaluate diet, and apply heat to muscles; also dorsiflex foot and press knee downward.

    h. Faintness: instruct to move slowly, avoid crowds, and remain in cool environment.

    i. Shortness of breath: encourage proper posture and use of pillows behind head and shoulders at night; instruct on rib cage lightening to increase flexibility of intercostal muscles.

    j. Difficulty sleeping: encourage a warm, caffeine-free drink before bed and use of relaxation techniques.

3. Help the couple deal with sexual changes and concerns.

4. Review the plan for labor and delivery, covering:

    a. Planned analgesia or anesthesia

    b. Breathing and relaxation methods

    c. Monitoring equipment

    d. Tour of labor and delivery area

    e. Plans for infant feeding

G. **Evaluation**

1. Maternal weight gain is within normal limits.

2. Fetal growth is within normal limits.

3. The patient exhibits no signs of complications.

4. The patient demonstrates positive adjustment to pregnancy.

5. The patient or couple exhibits adequate preparation for labor and delivery.

Bibliography

Danforth, D. N. (Ed.) (1986). *Obstetrics and gynecology* (5th ed.). Philadelphia: J. B. Lippincott.

Jensen, M. D., & Bobak, I. M. (1985). *Maternity and gynecologic care: The nurse and family* (3rd ed.). St. Louis: C. V. Mosby.

May, K. A., & Mahlmeister, L. R. (1990). *Comprehensive maternity nursing: Nursing process and the childbearing family* (2nd ed.). Philadelphia: J. B. Lippincott.

Olds, S. (1984). *Maternity-newborn nursing*. Menlo Park, CA: Addison-Wesley.

Reeder, S. J., & Martin, L. L. (1987). *Maternity nursing: Family, newborn, and women's health care* (16th ed.). Philadelphia: J. B. Lippincott.

STUDY QUESTIONS

1. Mary Smith arrives in the clinic for the first prenatal visit. The date of her last menstrual period was April 15. She asks the nurse "When is my baby due?" According to Nagele's rule, which of the following is the nurse's best response?
   a. January 29
   b. January 22
   c. February 29
   d. February 22

2. Mary asks the nurse how much she should gain during the pregnancy. The doctor told Mary she was underweight for her body build. The nurse's best response would be
   a. "You should gain 40 lb."
   b. "You should gain 15 lb."
   c. "You should gain 20 lb spread equally between the second and third trimesters."
   d. "You should gain 30 lb."

3. Mary confided in the nurse that she was afraid to have a baby because her sister had a complicated pregnancy. Which of the following is the best response for the nurse to give Mary?
   a. "Having a baby is safe these days."
   b. "Did you mention this to the doctor?"
   c. "This feeling is common; what specifically are you worried about?"
   d. "I wouldn't worry about it; your pregnancy will be different than your sister's."

4. Mary returned to the clinic at $4\frac{1}{2}$ months' gestation. Because of low hemoglobin, she was taking iron supplements and having dark stools and constipation. Based on this information, which of the following advice would the nurse give Mary?
   a. "This is common when taking iron."
   b. "I'll give you a list of foods that will alleviate your constipation."
   c. "The doctor may order a laxative such as Ex-Lax."

   d. "You could probably take an ounce of mineral oil to relieve constipation."

5. Mary returned to the clinic in 1 month, at $5\frac{1}{2}$ months' gestation. The urine evaluation indicated a trace of protein. The best response from the nurse would be which of the following?
   a. "A trace of protein is often common because of urinary changes in pregnancy."
   b. "The doctor may want to do a more extensive urinary study."
   c. "I'll talk to you about how to increase your fluid intake."
   d. "We want to really watch this so you don't develop complications."

6. The nurse explained to Mary that there are several danger signs that should be reported. These include all of the following *except*
   a. vaginal bleeding
   b. blurred vision
   c. leaking of amniotic fluid
   d. weight gain of 4 lb or more in 3 weeks

7. Mary explained to the nurse that she is a "real" coffee drinker—eight to 10 cups per day. Which of the following would be the nurse's best response?
   a. "Caffeine can cause congenital defects; therefore, we advise pregnant women to limit or avoid caffeine (coffee, tea, colas)."
   b. "If you drink caffeine after the first trimester, it is okay because most defects occur then."
   c. "You should reduce your caffeine consumption in half and you will probably be safe."
   d. "If you have 100 mg of caffeine per day, it is probably okay."

8. Mary returned at 32 weeks and complained of hemorrhoids. To assist with this problem, the nurse's best intervention would be to
   a. Instruct her to take sitz baths for 15 minutes three to four times daily.

b. Instruct her to talk to the physician about laxatives.

c. Instruct her to take a walk each day to help alleviate hemorrhoids.

d. Instruct her to talk to the physician about an exercise regimen.

9. Mary returned to the outpatient department at 7 months' gestation, complaining of heartburn. Which of the following instructions from the nurse would be most appropriate?

a. Take small sips of a carbonated drink, water, or milk.

b. Take small sips of ice water.

c. Take small sips of hot water.

d. Take Alka-Seltzer.

10. To assess most pelvic diameters, the nurse would usually place the patient in which of the following positions?

a. dorsal recumbent

b. knee–chest

c. lithotomy

d. Sim's

ANSWER KEY

1. **Correct response: b**
   According to Naegele's rule, one counts ahead 7 days and back 3 months.
   a, c, and d. These are all incorrect calculations.
   Application/Physiologic/Implementation

2. **Correct response: d**
   A weight gain of about 30 lb is average.
   a. A weight gain of 40 lb is excessive.
   b and c. A gain of 15 to 20 lb is insufficient unless the mother is overweight.
   Comprehensiven/Health promotion/ Implementation

3. **Correct response: c**
   This question helps the nurse identify specific problems and guide assessment.
   a. Pregnancy can become complicated even with good care.
   b. The nurse needs to handle this concern.
   d. The nurse should not disregard the patient's concern.
   Application/Psychosocial/Assessment

4. **Correct response: b**
   Proper diet is the safest way to alleviate constipation during pregnancy.
   a. This information is true but does not help the patient.
   c. Ex-Lax is a harsh laxative and should not be used.
   d. Mineral oil interferes with vitamin absorption and should not be used.
   Application/Safe care/Evaluation

5. **Correct response: a.**
   This is very common.
   b. This is not necessary.
   c. This was done before, and the patient is complying.
   d. This can cause guilt feelings when she is complying.
   Analysis/Safe care/Evaluation

6. **Correct response: d**
   Scales differ and need to be evaluated.
   a. This is a danger sign of abruptio placenta or placenta previa.
   b. This is a danger sign of pregnancy-induced hypertension.
   c. This is a danger sign of premature labor and increased chance of infection.
   Analysis/Health promotion/Implementation

7. **Correct response: a**
   Ideally, a woman should avoid caffeine during pregnancy.
   b. A pregnant woman should limit caffeine intake in all three trimesters of pregnancy.
   c and d. The safe level of caffeine intake during pregnancy is unknown.
   Application/Safe care/Implementation

8. **Correct response: a**
   Sitz baths are the safest way to treat hemorrhoids during pregnancy.
   b. Laxatives would not be ordered during pregnancy.
   c. The upright position of walking may aggravate the hemorrhoids.
   d. Exercise, although recommended during pregnancy, may aggravate hemorrhoids.
   Application/Safe care/Implementation

9. **Correct response: a**
   This will relieve heartburn.
   b and c. The patient should avoid hot and cold foods and fluids.
   d. This contains sodium and could cause fluid retention.
   Application/Safe care/Implementation

10. **Correct response: c**
    Pelvic examination is done primarily with the patient lying on her back with her legs in stirrups.
    a. In this position, the patient is lying flat on her back with her legs down.
    b. In this position, the patient is lying prone in a "jackknife" position (head and chest on table, buttocks in air, and knees on table).
    d. In this position, the patient is lying on her side with one knee flexed, placing the body in a semiprone position.
    Comprehensive/Physiologic/Implementation

Intrapartal Care

I. Overview

A. Intrapartal care

1. The intrapartal period extends from the beginning of contractions that cause cervical dilatation through delivery of the neonate and placenta and the first 1 to 4 hours after delivery.

2. Intrapartal care refers to the medical and nursing care given to a pregnant patient and family during labor and delivery.

B. Goals of intrapartal care

1. Promote maximum physical and emotional well-being in both the mother and the fetus.

99

2. Incorporate family-centered care concepts into the labor and delivery experience.

C. **Factors affecting the intrapartum experience**
   1. Previous experience with pregnancy
   2. Cultural and personal expectations
   3. Prepregnant health and biophysical preparedness for child-bearing
   4. Motivation for childbearing
   5. Socioeconomic readiness
   6. Age of mother; partnered versus unpartnered status; accessibility of prenatal care

D. **Nursing responsibilities**
   1. Determine maternal and fetal well-being on admission to the labor and delivery setting.
   2. Establish a welcoming environment that demonstrates to the client and and her family that quality care will be provided.
   3. Provide appropriate, clear, concise explanations about the physical surroundings, procedures, and expectations.
   4. Make timely, accurate assessments and interventions appropriate to the labor and delivery experience.

II. Phenomena and processes of labor and delivery

A. **Onset of labor**
   1. Labor is the process by which the fetus and products of conception are expelled as the result of regular, progressive, frequent, and strong uterine contractions.
   2. Labor initiation theories include:
      a. Progesterone deprivation
      b. Oxytocin stimulation
      c. Fetal endocrine control

B. **Factors affecting labor**
   1. *Passageway* refers to the pelvis and birth canal; factors include:
      a. Type of pelvis (e.g., gynecoid, android, anthropoid, platypelloid)
      b. Structure of pelvis (e.g., true vs. false pelvis)
      c. Pelvic inlet diameters
      d. Pelvic outlet diameters
      e. Ability of the uterine segment to distend, the cervix to dilate, and the vaginal canal and introitus to distend
   2. *Passenger* refers to the ability of the fetus to move through the passageway, based on:
      a. Size of the fetal head and capability of the head to mold to the passageway
      b. Fetal presentation, that part of the fetus that enters the maternal pelvis first (e.g., cephalic [vertex, face, brow], breech [frank, single or double footling, complete], shoulder [transverse lie])

    c.   Fetal attitude, the relationship of fetal parts to one another

    d.   Fetal position, the relationship of a particular reference point of the presenting part and the maternal pelvis, described with a series of three letters (i.e., side of maternal pelvis [L, left; R, right; T, transverse], presenting part [O, occiput; S, sacrum; Sc, scapula; M, mentum], and part of the maternal pelvis [A, anterior; P, posterior]; Fig. 9–1)

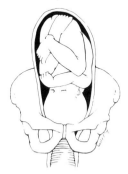

Left occipital posterior

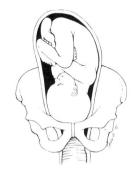

Left occipital transverse

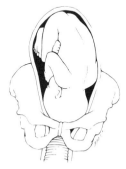

Left occipital anterior

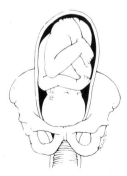

Right occipital posterior

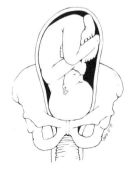

Right occipital transverse

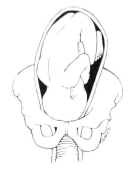

Right occipital anterior

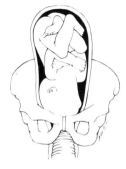

Left mentum anterior

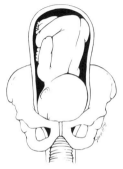

Right mentum posterior

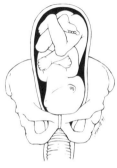

Right mentum anterior

FIGURE 9–1.
Fetal positions.

3. *Powers* refers to the frequency, duration, and strength of uterine contractions to cause complete cervical effacement and dilatation.
4. Placental factors involve the site of placental insertion.
5. *Psyche* refers to the patient's psychological state, available support systems, preparation for childbirth, past experiences, and coping strategies.

C. **Characteristics of true labor**
1. Contractions occur at regular intervals
2. Contractions start in the back and sweep around to the abdomen, increase in intensity and duration, with intervals that gradually shorten.
3. Contractions are intensified by walking.
4. "Bloody show" is usually present (pink-tinged mucus released from the cervical canal as labor starts).
5. Cervix becomes effaced and dilated.
6. Sedation does not stop contractions.

D. **Characteristics of false labor**
1. Contractions occur at irregular intervals
2. Located chiefly in abdomen, intensity remains the same, or is variable; intervals remain long.
3. Walking has no intensifying effect and often gives relief.
4. Bloody show is usually not present, or if present is usually brownish rather than bright red and may be due to recent pelvic examination or intercourse.
5. Cervix evidences no change.
6. Ambulation results in no change.
7. Sedation tends to decrease number of contractions.

E. **Signs and symptoms of impending labor (premonitory signs)**
1. Lightening: descent of the fetus and uterus into the pelvic cavity 2 to 3 weeks before onset of labor
2. Braxton Hicks contractions: irregular, intermittent contractions that have occurred during pregnancy become uncomfortable and produce a drawing pain in the abdomen and groin
3. Cervical changes: softening, "ripening," and effacement of the cervix will cause expulsion of the mucous plug (bloody show).
4. Rupture of membranes: amniotic membranes may rupture before the onset of labor.
5. Burst of energy or increased tension and fatigue
6. Weight loss of about 1 to 3 lb, 2 to 3 days before onset of labor

F. **Stages of labor**
1. First stage of labor
   a. Latent phase: begins with onset of regular contractions, effacement and dilatation of the cervix to 3 to 4 cm; lasts an average of 6.4 hours for nulliparas and 4.8 hours for

multiparas; contractions become increasingly stronger and more frequent.
    b. Active phase: dilatation continues from 3 to 4 cm to complete dilatation (10 cm); contractions become stronger, more frequent, longer in duration, and more painful. This active period is divided into three phases:
        (1) Acceleration phase
        (2) Phase of maximum slope
        (3) Deceleration or transition phase
    c. The interval between 8 and 10 cm dilatation also is referred to as the transition phase.
    d. The culmination of the active phase of labor is the deceleration phase (9 to 10 cm), when the mother feels more relaxed and perceives less discomfort, or the intensity, frequency, and duration of contractions may peak with an irresistible urge to push.

2. Second stage (expulsive stage)
    a. Begins with complete dilatation of cervix and ends with delivery of infant
    b. Contractions severe at 2- to 3-minute intervals, with a duration of 50 to 90 seconds
    c. Should be completed with in 1 hour after complete dilatation
    d. Infant is moved along birth canal by cardinal movements or mechanisms of labor (Fig. 9–2):
        (1) Descent
        (2) Flexion
        (3) Internal rotation
        (4) Extension
        (5) Restitution
        (6) External rotation
        (7) Expulsion
    e. "Crowning" occurs when infant's head or presenting part is at the vaginal opening.
    f. Episiotomy (surgical incision in perineum) may be done to facilitate delivery and avoid laceration of perineum.

3. Third stage (placenta stage)
    a. Begins with delivery of infant and ends with delivery of placenta
    b. Occurs in two phases: placental separation and placental expulsion
    c. Signs of placental separation: uterus becomes globular, fundus rises in abdomen, cord lengthens, and bleeding increases (trickle or gush).
    d. Contraction of the uterus controls uterine bleeding and aids with placental separation and expulsion.
    e. Oxytocic drugs are generally administered to help contract uterus.

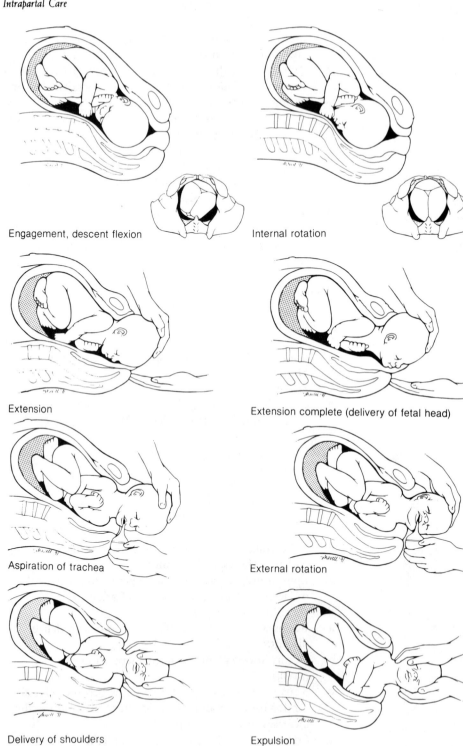

Engagement, descent flexion

Internal rotation

Extension

Extension complete (delivery of fetal head)

Aspiration of trachea

External rotation

Delivery of shoulders

Expulsion

FIGURE 9–2.
Cardinal Movements of Labor.

4. Fourth stage
    a. Involves delivery of placenta to 1 to 4 hours after birth and physiologic adjustment of patient's body to non-pregnant state
    b. Uterus contracts in midline of abdomen with fundus midway between umbilicus and symphysis pubis.

III. Essentials of intrapartal assessment

A. Maternal status and progress of labor

1. History: name, age, physician, weight, allergies, blood type and Rh, previous medical conditions, prenatal problems, gravida and para status, prenatal education, and method of infant feeding
2. Risk-factor screens: bleeding, premature rupture of membranes, hydramnios, abnormal presentation, multiple gestation, prolapsed cord, precipitous labor, meconium-stained amniotic fluid, fetal heart irregularities, postmaturity
3. Physiologic assessment:
    a. Maternal vital signs, weight, cardiac and respiratory status
    b. Fundal height
    c. Status of labor: contractions (onset, frequency, duration, intensity), membranes, bleeding, cervical dilatation, fetal descent
    d. Laboratory findings
4. Psychosocial status (e.g., anxiety, childbirth education, support systems, response to labor)
5. Evaluation of labor progress:
    a. Palpation or electronic monitoring (external with tocodynamometer and internal with intrauterine pressure catheter) to assess the phases, duration, frequency, and intensity of contractions
    b. Vaginal examination to assess cervical dilatation (opening of external os from closed to 10 mm) and cervical effacement (thinning and shortening of the cervix), as measured from 0% (thick) to 100% (paper thin) effaced
    c. Determination of station—the relationship of the presenting part to the pelvic ischial spines

B. Fetal assessment

1. Inspection of maternal abdomen to determine fetal lie—the relationship of the long axis (spine) of the fetus to the long axis of the mother; lies include:
    a. Longitudinal lie: long axis of fetus parallel to the long axis of the mother
    b. Transverse lie: long axis of fetus perpendicular to the long axis of the mother

2. Palpation of abdomen using the four Leopold maneuvers to determine fetal position and its possible size
3. Evaluation of fetal status
   a. Auscultation of fetal heart rate (FHR):
      (1) Normal range: 120 to 160 beats per minute
      (2) Decreases during contractions but returns to normal after 10 to 15 seconds
   b. Assessment of changes in FHR to identify:
      (1) Early deceleration: slowing of FHR early in contraction; considered benign
      (2) Late deceleration: indication of fetal hypoxia
      (3) Variable deceleration: transient decrease in FHR before, during, or after contraction; indication of cord compression
      (4) Bradycardia: FHR <100 beats per minute or a drop of 20 beats per minute below baseline; indication of cord compression or placental separation
      (5) Tachycardia: FHR >160 beats per minute; indication of fetal distress if persistent for over 1 hour or accompanied by late deceleration
      (6) Loss of baseline (beat-to-beat variability); indication of fetal demise
   d. Assessment of fetal acid–base status with fetal blood sampling or fetal scalp stimulation

IV. Intrapartal pain management
A. Overview of pain
1. Intrapartal pain refers to a subjective experience of the physical sensations associated with uterine contractions, cervical dilatation and effacement, and fetal descent during labor and birth.
2. Physiologic responses to pain may include increased blood pressure, pulse, respirations, perspiration, pupil diameter, muscle tension (facial tension, fisted hands) or muscle activity (e.g., pacing, turning, twisting)
3. Nonverbal expressions of pain may include withdrawal, hostility, fear, depression.
4. Verbal expression may include statements of pain, moaning, and groaning.
5. Pain relief may be achieved through prepared childbirth methods (e.g., Lamaze) analgesics, or regional anesthesia.
6. Intervention for pain relief during the intrapartal period depends on such factors as:
   a. Gestation
   b. Frequency, duration, and intensity of contractions
   c. Labor progress
   d. Maternal response to pain and labor
   e. Allergies and sensitivities to analgesics and anesthesia

B. Goals of pain management
1. Provide maximal relief of pain with maximal safety for mother and fetus.
2. Facilitate labor and delivery as a positive family experience.

C. Factors affecting perception of intrapartal pain
1. Previous experience with painful stimuli and personal expectations for the birth experience
2. Cultural concept of pain, specifically during childbirth, and how one should respond
3. Rapidly progressive uterine contractions
4. Fear and anxiety, fatigue

D. Pain theories (causes of intrapartal pain)
1. Uterine anoxia due to compressed muscle cells during contraction
2. Compression of the nerve ganglia in the cervix and lower uterine segment during contraction
3. Stretching of cervix during dilatation and effacement
4. Traction on, stretching and displacement of, the perineum.
5. Pressure on urethra, bladder, rectum during fetal descent
6. Distention of the lower uterine segment
7. Stretching of the uterine ligaments

E. Nursing responsibilities
1. Collaborate with mother and the birth attendant to determine the most effective method of pain relief during each stage and phase of the intrapartal period
2. Continually assess the mother's response to labor and the need for comfort, analgesia, or anesthesia
3. Continually assess fetal response to labor and pain-relief methods used

F. Nonpharmacologic pain-relief methods
1. Prepared childbirth methods can help the patient feel more in control and relaxed, helping her "work with" the contractions; may shorten labor.
2. Hypnosis may be useful in some patients
3. Interventions aimed at supporting the mother during labor may be helpful, such as:
   a. Providing information about the progress of labor
   b. Reinforcing techniques learned in prepared childbirth classes
   c. Instructing in breathing methods, abdominal lifting, pushing, relieving external pressure, distraction, cutaneous stimulation, and relaxation

G. Pharmacologic pain-relief methods
1. Analgesia
   a. Obstetric analgesia may include the use of analgesics (e.g., morphine, meperidine), sedative-hypnotics (e.g., barbiturates), or tranquilizers.

      b.   Analgesics provide very effective pain relief and slight sedation.

      c.   Maternal side effects include nausea, vomiting, mild respiratory depression, and transient mental impairment.

      d.   Analgesics are systemic drugs that readily cross the placental barrier, with depressive effects on the neonate occurring 2 to 3 hours after intramuscular injection.

      e.   Narcotic antagonists (i.e., Narcan) must be readily available in respiratory depression of mother or neonate

      f.   The decision to administer analgesia is predicated on the results of a vaginal examination; if birth is anticipated within 2 to 3 hours, the risk of neonatal narcosis may preclude the use of analgesics.

      g.   Dosages are kept to the smallest effective dose.

2. Barbiturates

      a.   These drugs cause maternal sedation and relaxation.

      b.   Maternal side effects of barbiturates include nausea, vomiting, hypotension, restlessness, and vertigo.

      c.   The rapid transfer of barbiturates across the placenta barrier and lack of an antagonist makes them generally inappropriate during active labor.

      d.   Newborn side effects of barbiturates include central nervous system depression, prolonged drowsiness, delayed establishment of feeding (e.g., due to poor sucking reflex or poor sucking pressure)

3. Tranquilizers

      a.   These drugs decrease the anxiety and apprehension associated with pain and sometimes relieve the nausea associated with analgesic use.

      b.   Tranquilizers potentiate active sedative and analgesic effects, decreasing the dosage needed to produce the desired effect.

      c.   Maternal side effects of tranquilizers include hypotension (which in turn decreases fetoplacental circulation), drowsiness, dizziness.

      d.   Fetal effects of tranquilizers include tachycardia and loss of normal beat-to-beat variability on electronic fetal heart monitoring.

      e.   Neonatal effects of tranquilizers include hypotonia, hypothermia, generalized drowsiness, and reluctance to feed for the first few days.

4. Regional anesthesia (conduction anesthesia)

      a.   Types include spinal block, epidural, paracervical, pudendal blocks and local infiltration.

      b.   These blocks provide pain relief by injecting anesthetic agents at sensory nerve pathways.

      c.   Adverse reactions may include maternal hypotension, al-

lergic or toxic reaction, respiratory paralysis, and partial
or total anesthetic failure.

    d.   Nursing responsibilities during administration of re-
gional anesthesia include assisting the anesthesiologist as
requested, establishing a reliable intravenous line, and
being prepared with medications and equipment for
emergency situations should they arise.

  5.   Systemic analgesics (e.g., narcotics, tranquilizers, seditives)
must be timed carefully to minimize effects on the fetus

  6.   Inhalation anesthesia (e.g., nitrous oxide, halothane) are used
rarely

  7.   General anesthesia (inhalant and intravenous) is used rarely in
labor and delivery

V. **Nursing management during first stage of labor**

  A. Assessment

    1.   Perform an initial assessment of labor status, covering:

      a.   Gravida and para status

      b.   Estimated date of delivery or estimated date of confine-
ment

      c.   Time of labor onset

      d.   Frequency and duration of contractions

      e.   Rupture of membranes, bloody show, or other signs of
labor onset

    2.   Assess maternal and fetal status, covering:

      a.   FHR

      b.   Status of amniotic membrane (if ruptured, note color)

      c.   Frequency, duration, and intensity of contractions

      d.   Maternal vital signs

      e.   Vaginal examination for cervical dilatation and efface-
ment, station and position of fetal presenting part

      f.   Maternal ability to cope with labor, available support
persons

  B. **Nursing diagnoses**

    1.   Ineffective Coping: Individual/Family

    2.   Fear

    3.   Fluid Volume Deficit

    4.   Knowledge Deficit

    5.   Altered Nutrition: Less than Body Requirements

    6.   Altered Oral Mucous Membranes

    7.   Self-care Deficit

    8.   Sleep Pattern Disturbance

    9.   Altered Tissue Perfusion

  C. **Planning and implementation**

    1.   On admission to the labor and delivery unit:

      a.   Collect urine specimen and order laboratory tests: he-

moglobin, hematocrit, serologic test for syphilis, and type and crossmatch (if indicated).
   b. Perform perineal preparation and enema, if indicated.
   c. Notify attending physician or midwife and report status.
   d. Provide support.
   e. Obtain informed consent from parturient.
2. During the first stage (latency phase):
   a. Provide information on emotional and physical support; provide pleasant, comfortable surroundings.
   b. Assess individual needs.
   c. Assess maternal temperature every 4 hours; if membranes ruptured, assess every hour.
   d. Assess blood pressure (BP), pulse, and respirations every hour. (If BP is > 140/90 or pulse is > 100, notify attending physician.)
   e. Assess uterine contractions (frequency, duration, and intensity) every 30 minutes.
   f. Assess FHR every 30 minutes.
   g. Assess cervical dilatation, effacement, station, and position of presenting part.
   h. Assess status of membranes; if ruptured, assess color of amniotic fluid. If membranes are ruptured and head is not at station 0, position mother to prevent cord prolapse.
   i. Interpret changes in the electronic fetal and maternal monitor strip and take appropriate action.
3. During the first stage, active phase:
   a. Provide safety, comfort, information, and emotional and physical support.
   b. Provide support during contractions: coach breathing, give back rubs, provide cool cloths.
   c. Assess contractions (frequency, duration, and intensity) every 15 to 30 minutes.
   d. Assess maternal blood pressure, pulse, and respirations every hour.
   e. Assess FHR every 15 minutes.
   f. Assess cervical dilatation, effacement, station, and position of presenting part as warranted.
   g. Provide pharmacologic support as indicated.
   h. Assess hydration status.
   i. Encourage voiding every 1 to 2 hours.
   j. Assess status of membranes; if ruptured, assess whether the presenting part is engaged. If not, check for prolapsed cord and position the patient accordingly.
   k. Interpret changes on the electronic fetal and maternal monitor strip and take appropriate action.
4. During the first stage, transition phase:

          a.   Provide information, comfort, and emotional and physical support.
          b.   Assess contractions (frequency, duration, and intensity) every 15 minutes.
          c.   Assess maternal blood pressure, pulse, and respirations every 30 minutes.
          d.   Assess FHR every 15 minutes.
          e.   Interpret changes on the electronic fetal and maternal monitor strip and take appropriate action if indicated.
          f.   Assess cervical dilatation, effacement, station, and position of presenting part; with complete dilatation, the fetus descends in the birth canal and the patient feels increased rectal pressure or the urge to push.

D. **Evaluation**
    1.   The pregnant patient progresses to complete dilatation.
    2.   The pregnant patient is able to begin pushing when completely dilated so as to aid decent of the presenting fetal part.
    3.   The patient's support system, nurses, and physician support her physically and emotionally to prepare for delivery.
    4.   The patient works effectively with contractions to facilitate delivery.
    5.   Vital signs, FHR remain within normal limits.
    6.   Hydration and elimination are adequate.
    7.   Staff is prepared for a sterile, controlled delivery.
    8.   Support person is physically and emotionally prepared.

VI. **Nursing management during second stage of labor**
  A. **Assessment**
    1.   Evaluate contractions for frequency, duration, and intensity (normal parameters include string contractions every 2 to 3 minutes, each lasting 45 to 90 seconds).
    2.   Monitor maternal blood pressure and pulse and FHR every 5 to 15 minutes.
    3.   Perform sterile vaginal examination to determine progress.
    4.   Interpret electronic fetal and maternal strip for changes

  B. **Nursing diagnoses**
    1.   High Risk for Ineffective Airway Clearance (neonate)
    2.   Ineffective Coping: Individual/Family (mother, other family members)
    3.   Fear (mother)
    4.   Fluid Volume Deficit (mother)
    5.   Hypothermia (neonate)
    6.   Knowledge Deficit (mother/family)
    7.   Altered Mucous Membranes (mother)
    8.   Pain (mother)
    9.   High Risk for Altered Parenting (family)
   10.   Self-care Deficit (mother)
   11.   Altered Tissue Perfusion (mother)

C. **Planning and implementation**

1. Notify physician or nurse midwife; provide emotional and physical support and comfort measures, and explain labor process and progress.
2. Assist the patient with pushing as indicated.
3. Prepare delivery area with equipment and supplies.
4. Prepare for delivery when perineal area is bulging in a primipara and when the cervix is dilated 7 to 8 cm in a multipara.
5. Place the patient in the birthing position.
6. Assist attending physician or nurse midwife with birth, help support person to be supportive, check all vital signs and FHR.
7. Establish and maintain a patent airway; suction with a bulb syringe or a DeLee mucus trap, and place the infant in modified Trendelenburg position on his or her side.
8. Compensate for poor neonatal thermoregulation by:
    a. Dry immediately with warm blanket.
    b. Place on radiant warmer.
    c. Wrap in warmed dry blanket or place in skin-to-skin contact with mother.
9. Obtain Apgar score at 1 and 5 minutes after delivery.
10. Inspect the umbilical cord for two arteries and one vein.
11. Weigh and measure the newborn as his or her condition stabilizes.
12. Footprint the newborn and fingerprint the mother.
13. Record the newborn's first voiding and stool passage.
14. Assess the newborn's gestational age.
15. Administer prophylactic eye medication to protect the conjunctivae from infection.
16. Administer Vitamin K (aquaMephyton) if ordered.

D. **Evaluation**

1. The patient verbalizes her understanding of the interventions use to promote comfort.
2. The patient verbalizes a decrease in her discomfort and shows signs of relaxing between explusive efforts.
3. The patient and support person verbalize a decrease in anxiety.
4. The patient uses effective breathing and expulsive techniques.
5. The patient assumes a position that facilitates expulsive efforts, maintains placental perfusion, and prevents or alleviates cord compression.
6. The newborn breathes spontaneously with a minimum of respiratory effort.
7. The newborn maintains skin temperature between 36.4°C and 37.2°C in the first hour after delivery.

VII. Nursing management during third stage of labor

A. Assessment

1. Evaluate maternal physiologic adjustment, covering such factors as:
   a. Vital signs
   b. Uterine firmness
2. Assess the new mother's emotional adjustment

B. Nursing diagnoses

1. Knowledge Deficit
2. Altered Oral Mucous Membranes
3. Pain
4. High Risk for Altered Parenting
5. Self-care Deficit

C. Planning and implementation

1. Promote physiologic adaptation by the new mother
2. Initiate fundal massage, gently, with adequate support to the lower uterine segment
3. Promote parent–infant interaction by placing the infant on the mother's abdomen and encouraging parents to touch the infant
4. Monitor mother and newborn for potential complications
5. Document intrapartal care; for example:
   a. Time of delivery of infant and placenta
   b. 1- and 5-minute Apgar scores
   c. Any immediate neonatal care provided
   d. Extent and repair of perineal lacerations or episiotomy
   e. Estimated maternal blood loss
   f. Medications administered before, during, and after delivery (to mother and neonate)
   g. Placement of identification bands; footprinting and fingerprinting
   h. Maternal and fetal vital signs

D. Evaluation

1. Maternal bleeding is within normal limits with firm uterine tone and normal maternal vital signs.
2. The new mother verbalizes comfort with fundal massage.
3. Parents and newborn begin interaction by intent face-to-face gazing and parental exploration of infant.
4. Complications, if any, are promptly identified and appropriate action taken.
5. Documentation of intrapartal care is accurate and complete.

Bibliography

Danforth, D. N. (Ed.) (1986). *Obstetrics and gynecology* (5th ed.). Philadelphia: J. B. Lippincott.

Jensen, M. D., & Bobak, I. M. (1985). *Maternity and gynecologic care: The nurse and family* (3rd ed.). St. Louis: C. V. Mosby.

May, K.A., & Mahlmeister, L. R. (1990). *Comprehensive maternity nursing: Nursing process and the childbearing family* (2nd ed.). Philadelphia: J. B. Lippincott.

Olds, S. (1984). *Maternity-newborn nursing.* Menlo Park, CA: Addison-Wesley.

Reeder, S. J., & Martin, L. L. (1987). *Maternity nursing: Family, newborn, and women's health care* (16th ed.). Philadelphia: J. B. Lippincott.

STUDY QUESTIONS

1. The nurse explains to Mary and John the purpose of effleurage. Which of the following would be the best explanation?
   a. This is massage of the legs to remove cramps that occur during labor.
   b. This is gentle massage of the abdomen to facilitate relaxation.
   c. This is what we call application of pressure over the sacral area to relieve backache.
   d. This is a form of biofeedback for relaxation.

2. If a laboring woman breathes improperly when using a method of childbirth preparation, the result could be which of the following?
   a. increased pulse
   b. hyperventilation
   c. hypertension
   d. fetal heart rate decelerations

3. The method of childbirth preparation that is based on the fear-tension-pain mechanism is which of the following?
   a. Lamaze
   b. Dick-Read
   c. Bradley
   d. Kitzinger

4. Labor is divided into stages. The first stage of labor is completed when
   a. The baby is delivered.
   b. The cervix is completely dilated.
   c. Labor becomes more intense.
   d. The placenta is delivered.

5. An important assessment that is conducted during labor is the fetal heart rate. Which of the following is a normal fetal heart rate range?
   a. 100 to 120 beats per minute

   b. 120 to 160 beats per minute
   c. 150 to 180 beats per minute
   d. 100 to 140 beats per minute

6. The nurse performs Leopold's maneuvers for which one of the following purposes?
   a. to diagnose fetal well-being
   b. to determine fetal heart tones
   c. to determine cervical dilatation
   d. to determine fetal position and presentation

7. Which of the following fetal positions is the most common for delivery?
   a. left occiput anterior
   b. left occiput posterior
   c. left sacral anterior
   d. right sacral posterior

8. If the baby is in the proper position for delivery, which of the following fetal head structures will the nurse be able to feel on digital vaginal examination at 6 cm dilatation and station 0?
   a. anterior fontanel and frontal suture
   b. coronal suture
   c. posterior fontanel
   d. lambdoidal suture

9. A patient calls the delivery room and asks the characteristics of *true* contractions. Which of the following would be the nurse's best response?
   a. True contractions begin in the lower abdomen.
   b. True contractions are difficult to determine because they come and go.
   c. True contractions have a regularity and become more intense over time.
   d. True contractions decrease with activity.

ANSWER KEY

1. *Correct response: b*
This facilitates relaxation and takes concentration.
  a. Flexion of the foot may relieve leg cramps.
  c. Application of pressure has no specific name.
  d. Biofeedback may produce relaxation, but this is not effleurage.
Application/Psychological/Implementation

2. *Correct response: b*
Improper breathing patterns commonly cause hyperventilation during labor.
  a. This may occur but is not the best answer.
  c. Blood pressure should not be affected.
  d. Contractions and maternal position affect fetal heart rate.
Comprehension/Physiologic/Analysis

3. *Correct response: b*
Grantly Dick-Read advanced the concept of fear-tension-pain mechanism.
  a. Lamaze includes exercise, relaxation, breathing, nutrition, infant feeding, sexuality, parenting, and coping with postpartum.
  c. This is called husband-coached and emphasizes slow, deep breathing and deep relaxation.
  d. Teaches the use of sensory memory to understand and work with one's body in preparation for birth.
Knowledge/Psychological/Analysis

4. *Correct response: b*
Complete cervical dilatation marks the end of the first stage of labor.
  a. This is the second stage.
  c. This occurs during the first stage.
  d. This occurs during the third stage.
Knowledge/Physiologic/Assessment

5. *Correct response: b*
Normal fetal heart rate ranges from 120 to 160 beats per minute.

a and d. These rates are much too slow.
  c. This rate is much too fast.
Knowledge/Physiologic/Assessment

6. *Correct response: d*
Leopold's maneuvers help the nurse determine fetal lie and presentation.
  a. Sonogram will determine fetal well-being.
  b. Fetoscope and doptone determine fetal heart tones.
  c. Cervical dilatation is determined by digital vaginal examination.
Application/Health promotion/Assessment

7. *Correct response: a*
This is the most common position and usually does not require forceps.
  b. This is completely turned, coined a "sunny-side-up" baby (face first); often they have problems.
  c and d. Baby will probably need low forceps or, depending on fetal flexion, a cesarean delivery.
Application/Physiologic/Planning

8. *Correct response: a*
The anterior fontanel and frontal suture can be felt when the baby is in the proper position in the birth canal.
  b. The coronal suture is to the side of the fetal head.
  c. The posterior fontanel is toward the back of the head.
  d. The lamboidal suture is behind the posterior fontanel.
Analysis/Physiologic/Assessment

9. *Correct response: c*
True contractions occur in a regular pattern and increase in intensity as labor progresses.
  a. True contractions usually begin in the lower back.
  b. This does not answer the question.
  d. This is not a complete answer.
Application/Safe care/Implementation

Postpartal Care

I. Overview

A. Essential concepts

1. Postpartum care refers to the medical and nursing care given to a patient from the time of delivery until her body returns to near its nonpregnant state.

2. The puerperium is the 6-week period after delivery, beginning with termination of labor and ending with the return of the reproductive organs to the nonpregnant state; a physical and psychological adjustment to the process of childbearing.

3. Involution refers to the progressive changes in the uterus after delivery, leading to its return to prepregnant size and condition.

      4.   This period is sometimes referred to as the fourth trimester of pregnancy.

      5.   One aspect of care that commonly suffers with the trend toward earlier discharge is support in breast-feeding.

B. **Goals of postpartal care**

      1.   Promote normal involution and return to the nonpregnant state.

      2.   Prevent or minimize postpartum complications.

      3.   Promote comfort and healing of pelvic, perianal, and perineal tissues.

      4.   Assist in restoration of normal body functions.

      5.   Increase understanding of physiologic and psychological changes.

      6.   Facilitate newborn care and self-care by the new mother.

      7.   Promote the newborn's successful integration into the family unit.

      8.   Support parenting skills and parent–infant attachment.

      9.   Provide effective discharge planning, including appropriate referral for home care follow-up.

C. **Factors affecting the postpartal experience**

      1.   Nature of labor and delivery and the birth outcome

      2.   Preparation for labor and delivery and for parenting

      3.   Abruptness of the transition to parenthood

      4.   Family's individual and collective experiences with childbearing and childrearing

      5.   Family members' role expectations

      6.   Sensitivity and effectiveness of nursing and other professional care

      7.   Factors that increase the risk of postpartum complications include:

         a.   Preeclampsia or eclampsia

         b.   Diabetes

         c.   Cardiac problems

         d.   Uterine overdistention (e.g., due to multiple births or hydramnios)

         e.   Abruptio placenta or placenta previa

         f.   Precipitous or prolonged labor, difficult delivery, extended period of time spent in stirrups

D. **Nursing responsibilities**

      1.   Provide sensitive professional care to the new parents, which includes:

         a.   Accurate assessment of mother's physiologic and psychological status

         b.   Anticipatory guidance and health teaching as needed

      2.   Facilitate the family's bonding experience

II. Postpartal biophysical changes

A. Reproductive system changes

1. The *uterus* contracts firmly, reducing its size by over one half; it remains this size for about 2 days, then decreases in size (involution) and descends about one finger-breadth per day.

2. At 10 to 14 days postpartum, the uterus cannot be palpated abdominally. It returns to its nonpregnant size by 4 to 6 weeks' postpartum. The site of placental attachment requires 6 to 7 weeks to heal; endometrial regeneration requires 6 weeks.

3. *Lochia*, discharge from the uterus during the first 3 weeks following delivery, occurs in three types:

    a. Lochia rubia: dark red discharge in the first 2 to 3 days, containing epithelial cells, erythrocytes, leukocytes, and decidua

    b. Lochia serosa: pink to brownish discharge seen from day 3 to day 10 after delivery; serosanguineous discharge containing decidua, erythrocytes, leukocytes, cervical mucus, and microorganisms

    c. Lochia alba: almost colorless to creamy yellowish discharge, occurring from 10 days to 3 weeks after delivery and containing leukocytes, decidua, epithelial cells, fat, cervical mucus, cholesterol crystals, and bacteria

4. The *cervix* becomes thicker and firmer; by the end of the first postpartal week, it is still dilated about 1 cm. Complete cervical involution may take 3 to 4 months; childbirth results in a permanent change in the cervical os from round to elongated.

5. The *vagina* is smooth and swollen, with poor tone after delivery. Rugae reappear by 3 to 4 weeks postpartum, and estrogen index returns in 6 to 10 weeks.

6. The *perineum* appears edematous and bruised after delivery; episiotomy or lacerations may be present.

7. The *abdomen* remains soft and flabby for some time after delivery. Striae remain, but take on a silvery-white appearance. Diastasis recti (separation of abdominal recti muscles) may occur in women with poor muscle tone.

8. *Breast* changes include:

    a. Rapid drop in estrogen and progesterone levels with an increase in secretion of prolactin after delivery

    b. Colostrum present at time of delivery; breast milk produced by the third or fourth postpartum day

    c. Breasts becoming larger and firmer as lactation is established (primary engorgement), with this congestion subsiding in 1 or 2 days

9. In the breast, prolactin stimulates alveolar cells to produce milk. Sucking of newborn causes oxytocin release and contractility of myoepithelial cells to stimulate milk flow, known as the let-down

reflex. The average amount of milk produced in 24 hours increases over time:
    a.   First week: 6 to 10 oz
    b.   1 to 4 weeks: 20 oz
    c.   After 4 weeks: 30 oz

B. **Endocrine system changes**
    1.   Estrogen and progesterone levels decrease rapidly after delivery.
    2.   Ovulation and return of menstruation are influenced by whether or not a the patient breast-feeds.
        a.   Lactating: 45% of women resume menstruation by 12 weeks; 80% have one or more anovulatory cycles before the first ovulation.
        b.   Nonlactating: 40% of women resume menstruation by 6 weeks after delivery, 65% by 12 weeks, and 90% by 24 weeks; 50% ovulate during the first cycle.
    3.   A rapid drop in estrogen and progesterone following delivery of the placenta is responsible for many of the anatomic and physiologic changes in the puerperium.
    4.   Requirements for rest and sleep increase significantly.

C. **Cardiovascular system changes**
    1.   Transient bradycardia (40 to 70 beats per minute) occurs for 24 to 48 hours after delivery and may persist for the first 6 to 8 days.
    2.   Blood volume decreases to nonpregnant levels by 2 weeks after delivery.
    3.   Hematocrit rises by the third to seventh postpartum day.
    4.   Leukocytosis (20,000 to 25,000 white blood cells/mL) continues for several days after delivery to prevent infection.
    5.   Blood pressure remains stable; pulse returns to nonpregnant rate by 3 months postpartum.

D. **Respiratory system changes: pulmonary functions return to nonpregnant status by 6 months after delivery.**

E. **Renal and urinary system changes**
    1.   Overdistention of the bladder is common due to increased bladder capacity, swelling, bruising of tissues around the urethra, and diminished sensation to increased pressure.
    2.   A full bladder will displace the uterus and can cause postpartum hemorrhage; bladder distention can lead to urinary retention.
    3.   Adequate bladder emptying generally resumes in 5 to 7 days after tissue swelling and bruising resolve.
    4.   Glomerular filtration rate remains elevated for about 7 days after delivery.
    5.   Dilated ureters and renal pelvis return to their nonpregnant states in 6 to 10 weeks after delivery.
    6.   Puerperal diaphoresis and diuresis occur within the first 24 hours after delivery.

F. Gastrointestinal (GI) system changes
   1. Hunger and thirst are common after delivery.
   2. GI motility and tone return to the nonpregnant state within 2 weeks after delivery.
   3. Constipation commonly occurs during the early postpartum period.
   4. The patient may return to her prepregnant weight in 6 to 8 weeks if weight gain during pregnancy was within the normal range.
   5. Hemorrhoids are a common problem in the early postpartal period, due to pressure on the pelvic floor and straining during labor.

G. Musculoskeletal system changes
   1. Most women ambulate 4 to 8 hours after delivery; early ambulation is encouraged to avoid complications, promote involution, and improve emotional outlook.
   2. Relaxation and increased mobility of pelvic articulations occur 6 to 8 weeks after delivery.

H. Integumentary system changes
   1. Melanin decreases gradually after delivery, causing decrease in hyperpigmentation (coloration may not return to prepregnant status, however).
   2. Visible vascular changes of pregnancy disappear as estrogen levels decrease.

III. Postpartal psychosocial adaptation
   A. Essential concepts
   1. The postpartal period represents a time of emotional stress for the new mother, made even more difficult by the tremendous physiologic changes that occur.
   2. Factors influencing successful transition to parenthood during the postpartal period include:
      a. Response and support of family and friends
      b. Relationship of the birthing experience to expectations and aspirations
      c. Previous childbearing and childrearing experiences
      d. Cultural influences
   3. This period is described by Rubin as occurring in three stages: taking in, taking hold, and letting go.

   B. Taking-in period
   1. During this period, occurring 1 to 2 days after delivery, the new mother typically is passive and dependent, with energies focused on bodily concerns.
   2. She may review her labor and delivery experience frequently.
   3. Uninterrupted sleep is important if the mother is to avoid the effects of sleep deprivation—fatigue, irritability, interference with normal restorative processes.

4. Additional nourishment may be needed, because the mother's appetite is usually increased; poor appetite may be a clue that the restorative process is not progressing normally.

C. Taking-hold period

1. During this period, extending from 2 to 4 days after delivery, the mother becomes concerned with her ability to parent successfully, and accepts increasing responsibility for her infant.

2. The mother focuses on regaining control over her body functions—bowel and bladder function, strength, and endurance.

3. The mother strives to master infant-care skills (e.g., holding, breast- or bottle-feeding, bathing, diapering). She may be sensitive to feelings of inadequacy in this area and may tend to perceive the nurse's suggestions as overt or covert criticism. The nurse should take this into account when providing patient teaching and emotional support.

D. Letting-go period

1. This period generally occurs after the new mother returns home; it involves a time of family reorganization.

2. The mother assumes responsibility for newborn care; she must adapt to demands of the infant's dependency as well as to her decreased autonomy, independence, and (typically) social interaction.

3. Postpartum depression most commonly occurs during this period.

E. Postpartum depression

1. Many mothers experience a "let-down" feeling after giving birth, related to the magnitude of the birth experience and doubts about the ability to cope effectively with the demands of childrearing.

2. Typically, this depression is mild and transient, beginning 2 to 3 days after delivery and resolving within 1 to 2 weeks.

3. Rarely, relatively mild depression leads to postpartum psychosis, a pathologic condition.

IV. Nursing management during the normal postpartal period

A. Assessment

1. Focus ongoing assessment on early identification of and prompt intervention for complications.

2. During the critical first hour after delivery, carefully assess for hemorrhage, checking the fundus frequently, inspecting the perineum for visible bleeding, and evaluating vital signs.

3. On subsequent postpartal assessments, include vital signs, fundus, lochia, perineum, breasts, elimination, nutrition, ambulation and exercise, rest and sleep patterns, and self-care and infant care.

4. Vital signs: assess temperature, blood pressure, pulse, and respi-

rations every 4 to 8 hours during the first few days postpartum; note especially:

    a. Mild temperature elevation, which may be due to dehydration, onset of lactation, or leukocytosis

    b. Hypotension with rapid thready pulse (<100), which may signify hemorrhage and shock

    c. Orthostatic hypotension due to cardiovascular readjustment to the nonpregnant state

    d. Elevated blood pressure, possibly indicating pregnancy-induced hypertension

5. Assess the fundus daily for firmness and location; make sure the patient empties her bladder before palpating. Look for indications of subinvolution:

    a. Uterus not progressively decreasing in size or returning to the lower pelvis

    b. Uterus remaining flabby and poorly contracted

    c. Persistent backache or pelvic pain

    d. Heavy vaginal bleeding

6. Assess the amount and character of lochia daily to provide an essential index of endometrial healing. Report any abnormal findings, such as:

    a. Fresh bleeding

    b. Heavy, persistent, and malodorous lochia rubra

7. Inspect the perineum, noting status of sutures (if present), tenderness, swelling, bruising, and hematoma; assess anal area for hemorrhoids and fissures.

8. Assess breasts for firmness, tenderness, and warmth, and nipples for cracks, fissures, and bleeding; handle breasts gently.

9. Evaluate the patient's level of knowledge about infant feeding (breast- and bottle-feeding).

10. Assess degree of bladder distension often in the first 8 hours after delivery. Monitor urine output; voiding small amounts on frequent consecutive voidings indicates residual urine and possible need for catheterization.

11. Assess status of bowel elimination and the return to predelivery patterns.

12. Evaluate nutritional status, including ability to ingest food and fluids and adequacy of diet to support involution and lactation.

13. Assess ambulation, rest and exercise patterns, and ability to perform activities of daily living.

14. Assess peripheral circulation, noting varicosities, edema, and symmetry of size and shape, temperature, color, and range of motion. Note particularly signs of thrombophlebitis, positive Homan's sign.

15. Assess psychosocial adaptation, including:

    a. Signs and symptoms of postpartum "blues": crying, despondency, loss of appetite, poor concentration, difficulty sleeping, anxiety

    b. Evaluate integration of the newborn into the family.

    c. Observe interactions of the new mother and other family members with the infant.

B. **Nursing diagnoses**

1. Anxiety
2. Body Image Disturbance
3. Constipation
4. High Risk for Infection
5. High Risk for Injury
6. Knowledge Deficit
7. Pain
8. Altered Parenting
9. Altered Role Performance
10. Self-care Deficit
11. Sexual Dysfunction
12. Altered Patterns of Urinary Elimination

C. **Planning and implementation**

1. Teach the new mother aspects of self-care and newborn care.
2. Observe the new mother providing care for her newborn.
3. Report and record increased pulse rate, decreased blood pressure, and elevated temperature.
4. Gently massage the fundus if baggy; express clots from the fundus as indicated.
5. Apply ice or cold therapy to the episiotomy or lacerations immediately after delivery to decrease edema and provide anesthesia; thereafter, apply moist or dry heat therapy to promote comfort and healing.
6. Apply anesthetic sprays, ointments, or witch hazel pads to the perineum to promote comfort; administer analgesia as ordered and indicated; provide sitz baths as needed.
7. Instruct the patient on sitting properly to relieve pain: squeeze buttocks together and contract pelvic floor muscles before sitting. Also instruct her to wear perineal pads loosely and to lie in Sim's position.
8. Teach the patient to cleanse her breasts daily, with clean water if breast-feeding and with soap and water if bottle-feeding, and to wear a well-fitting brassiere.
9. Treat breast pain with analgesics and ice packs.
10. Assist with breast-feeding, as needed; explain mechanisms involved in lactation, breast care, positioning of self and infant, and nursing techniques.
11. Encourage the patient to void within first 4 to 8 hours after delivery and every 2 to 3 hours thereafter. If necessary, help stimulate

urination by running water, placing her hands in warm water, giving warm beverage, providing privacy and support, or pouring warm water over the vulva.

12. Teach the patient to cleanse the perineum after each voiding and defecation, wiping from front to back, then to wash her hands and apply a perineal pad also from front to back.

13. Provide adequate dietary fiber and fluids to promote bowel movements; if necessary, administer stool softeners, laxatives, suppositories, or enemas. Teach the importance of good fluid intake, exercise, proper diet, and establishing a regular defecation time.

14. Ensure good nutrition and fluid intake.

15. Support the patient's attempts at ambulation and exercise; explain the advantages of early ambulation and regular exercise in preventing complications and strengthening muscles of the back, pelvic floor, and abdomen.

16. Instruct the patient to avoid garters or constricting clothing that can impair circulation.

17. Limit visitors and adjust hospital routine to enable adequate rest.

18. Permit the patient to shower as soon as she can ambulate, and to take tub baths after 2 weeks. Recommend a daily shower to promote comfort and a sense of well-being.

19. Provide emotional and psychological support during the transition to parenthood, including:

    a. Encouraging the mother to hold and explore her new infant

    b. Facilitating visitation by partner and others

    c. Providing time for parent–infant contact, as indicated by the mother's and infant's condition

    d. Explaining postpartal hormonal changes and how they can affect emotions and mood

    e. Teaching infant care and safety measures

    f. Providing analgesia and position changes for comfort and promoting adequate rest; stressing the need for adequate rest to enhance coping ability

    g. Discussing expected infant developmental milestones and expected maternal physical and psychological changes in the postpartal period

    h. Discussing resumption of sexual activity—typically, intercourse can be safely resumed after 3 weeks; other forms of sexual expression need not be affected

    i. Explaining the newborn's need to be touched, held, and spoken to often; discuss the infant's response to various stimuli

    j. Encouraging the new parents to express feelings and concerns

20. Encourage the patient to schedule a 6-week check-up to assess her general physical condition, progress of involution, and family adaptation to the newborn.

D. Evaluation
   1. During the immediate postpartal period:
      a. The patient exhibits normal uterine involution.
      b. Vital signs, weight, and healing of episiotomy are within accepted parameters.
      c. The patient requests and tolerates food and fluids.
      d. The patient empties bladder as needed.
      e. The patient rests well between procedures and observations.
      f. The patient holds and explores infant.
   2. During postpartum hospitalization:
      a. Vital signs, weight, breasts, involutional process, and healing of episiotomy are within expected parameters.
      b. The patient maintains bowel and bladder elimination.
      c. The patient performs breast and perineal care.
      d. The patient rests and sleeps well.
      e. The patient verbalizes correct self-care and newborn care.
   3. In preparation for discharge:
      a. The patient demonstrates satisfactory infant care ability.
      b. The patient verbalizes the importance of follow-up care for herself and her infant.
      c. The patient knows how to contact primary physician, obstetrician, pediatrician, midwife, primary nurse.
      d. The patient expresses understanding of psychosocial needs of the newborn and parent-sibling-family interaction.
      e. The couple verbalizes understanding of changes in sexual response, when they can safely resume intercourse, and the use of contraception.
   4. At the 6-week check-up:
      a. Vital signs—weight, breast changes, involutional process, and healing of episiotomy—are within expected parameters.
      b. The patient's reproductive organs return to prepregnant condition.
      c. The family demonstrates positive adaptation and function.
      d. The couple meets their contraceptive goal.

Bibliography

Brunner, L. S., & Suddarth, D. S. (1987). *The Lippincott manual of nursing practice* (4th ed.). Philadelphia: J. B. Lippincott.

Danforth, D. N. (Ed.) (1986). *Obstetrics and gynecology* (5th ed.). Philadelphia: J. B. Lippincott.

Jensen, M. D., & Bobak, I. M. (1985). *Maternity and gynecologic care: The nurse and family* (3rd ed.). St. Louis: C. V. Mosby.

May, K. A., & Mahlmeister, L. R. (1990). *Comprehensive maternity nursing: Nursing process and the childbearing family* (2nd ed.). Philadelphia: J. B. Lippincott.

Olds, S. (1984). *Maternity-newborn nursing*. Menlo Park, CA: Addison-Wesley.

Reeder, S. J., & Martin, L .L. (1987). *Maternity nursing: Family, newborn, and women's health care* (16th ed.). Philadelphia: J. B. Lippincott.

STUDY QUESTIONS

1. The nurse told Ms. May that many changes occur during the puerperium. Ms. May asked, "What is the puerperium?" Which of the following would be the nurse's best response? The puerperium is
   a. a 4- to 6-hour period after delivery during which the placenta is completely expelled.
   b. a phase of the fourth stage of labor
   c. a term to indicate progressive changes of the breast 4 to 6 weeks after delivery
   d. a 6-week period after delivery, during which the reproductive organs return to a nonpregnant state

2. On the second day after delivery, the lochia discharge should be marked by which of the following?
   a. contain large clots
   b. lochia serosa
   c. lochia alba
   d. lochia rubra

3. Ellen, a gravida 1 para 1, delivered a 7-lb male infant. She plans to breast-feed. On the first postpartum day, the nurse notes that Ellen's fundus is above the umbilicus and to the left of the midline. What would the nurse initially suspect?
   a. a full bladder
   b. retained placental fragments
   c. uterine atony
   d. uterine inertia

4. Ellen complains of tenderness and swelling of her breasts. The nurse explains that she is experiencing primary breast engorgement, which should last for
   a. 1 to 2 days
   b. 3 to 4 days
   c. 5 to 6 days
   d. 7 to 8 days

5. To keep the nipples in good condition for breast-feeding and to prevent the potential for infection, which of the following would the nurse teach Ellen to include in her daily care?
   a. Wash with soap and water before each feeding.
   b. Keep the nipples dry and clean.
   c. Cover the nipples with a dry and clean plastic pad.
   d. Cleanse with antiseptic solution three times a day.

6. Ellen is disturbed because she needs to void large amounts of urine frequently. How would the nurse best respond to Ellen? Urinating large amounts frequently
   a. is a sign of urinary retention and overflow
   b. is normal because it reduces extracellular fluid acquired during pregnancy
   c. is a result of decreased bladder tone due to anesthesia during labor
   d. is an indication of a bladder infection

7. Ellen asks, "When will the stretch marks on my abdomen and breasts disappear?" What would be the nurse's best response to Ellen? The stretch marks will
   a. disappear in 4 to 6 weeks
   b. disappear if you use a vitamin ointment
   c. fade and become silvery white in color
   d. not disappear

8. Ellen is dismissed on her third postpartum day. What type of lochia should be noted?
   a. lochia alba
   b. lochia serosa
   c. lochia rubra
   d. lochia rugae

9. What type of vaginal discharge would Ellen demonstrate 2 weeks after delivery in the outpatient clinic?
   a. lochia alba
   b. lochia serosa
   c. lochia rubra
   d. lochia sanguineous

10. What is used to relieve perineal discomfort on the second postpartum day?
    a. application of ice bags

b. application of heat

c. administration of oxytocin

d. administration of hormones

11. If the fundus of the uterus is felt at the umbilicus immediately after delivery of the placenta, the nurse should take which one of the following nursing actions?

a. Catheterize the patient.

b. Massage the fundus to make it firm.

c. Administer Methergine.

d. Support the mother, because this represents normal fundus placement.

ANSWER KEY

1. **Correct response: d**
   The puerperium is a 6-week period after delivery during which the female reproductive organs return to a nonpregnant state.
   a, b, and c. None of these responses describes the puerperium.
   Comprehension/Safe care/Implementation

2. **Correct response: d**
   Two days after delivery the discharge is bright red.
   a. If discharge has large clots, she is bleeding too heavily.
   b. Lochia serosa occurs about 5 to 7 days after delivery.
   c. Lochia rubra occurs about day 10 after delivery.
   Comprehension/Safe care/Implementation

3. **Correct response: a**
   A full bladder will displace the uterus up on the abdomen and to either side of the midline.
   b. With retained placental fragments, the woman would complain of excessive cramping, and there would be a large amount of lochia.
   c. With uterine atony, the uterus would not contract properly and would be baggy.
   d. Uterine inertia is the inability of the uterus to contract during labor.
   Comprehension/Safe care/Implementation

4. **Correct response: a**
   Primary breast engorgement is caused by stasis of blood and lymph in the breasts and will last 1 to 2 days.
   b, c, and d. These fine frames are all incorrect; breast engorgement persisting longer than 1 to 2 days necessitates further investigation.
   Comprehension/Safe care/Implementation

5. **Correct response: b**
   It is important to keep the nipples clean and dry so that they do not crack and become infected.
   a. Washing with soap and water before each feeding will cause the nipples to become dry and cracked.
   c. If the nipples and areola are covered with plastic breast pads, moisture will accumulate and cause bacteria to grow, thus predisposing to breast infection.
   d. Cleansing with an antiseptic solution will cause the nipples to become dry and cracked.
   Comprehension/Safe care/Implementation

6. **Correct response: b**
   Diuresis is normal. It is a reaction that acts to reduce extracellular fluid acquired during pregnancy.
   a. Frequent voiding of small amounts is a sign of urinary retention and overflow.
   c. With decreased bladder tone, there would be inability to void.
   d. With a bladder infection, there would be frequency and burning.
   Comprehension/Safe care/Implementation

7. **Correct response: c**
   The striae will eventually fade to a silvery white color.
   a. Fading of striae occurs gradually and will take longer than 4 to 6 weeks.
   b. The use of vitamin ointment will not enhance the fading of the striae.
   d. The striae will fade over time.
   Comprehension/Safe care/Implementation

8. **Correct response: c**
   Lochia rubra is seen 1 to 3 days postpartum.
   a. Lochia alba is seen 1 to 3 weeks postpartum.
   b. Lochia serosa is seen 5 to 7 days postpartum.
   d. There is no lochia rugae.
   Comprehension/Safe care/Implementation

9. **Correct response: a**

Lochia alba is seen 1 to 3 weeks postpartum.

b. Lochia serosa is seen 5 to 7 days postpartum.

c. Lucia rubra is seen 1 to 3 days postpartum.

d. There is no lochia sanguineous.

Comprehension/Safe care/Implementation

10. *Correct response: b*

Moist or dry heat is applied to the perineal area for discomfort after the first postpartum day, because it will increase circulation and enhance healing.

a. Ice bags are applied to the perineal area in the first few hours after delivery to decrease discomfort and edema.

c. Oxytocic is administered to contract the uterus.

d. Hormones are not indicated for perineal discomfort.

Comprehension/Safe care/Implementation

11. *Correct response: b*

The fundus should be midway between umbilicus and pubis.

a. Catheterization is not done unless absolutely necessary because of the increased chance of infection.

c. Pitocin is drug of choice after delivery because it causes sustained contraction.

d. This is not proper location.

Application/Safe care/Evaluation

Newborn Care

I. Overview

A. Essential concepts

1. In the postpartal period, the newborn experiences complex biophysiologic and behavior changes related to the transition to extrauterine life.

2. Nursing care of the newborn is based on knowledge of these changes and of the newborn's impact on the family unit.

3. The first few hours after birth represent a critical period of adjust-

ment for the newborn. In most settings, the nurse provides direct care to the newborn immediately after birth.

4. After the transition period, the nurse continues to evaluate the newborn at periodic intervals and to alter nursing care plans according to ongoing findings.

5. The nurse must be skillful in balancing the family's need for privacy and time to interact without interruptions with the need to closely monitor the newborn's transition to extrauterine life.

B. Goals of newborn care

1. For the initial postpartal period
   a. Establish and maintain an airway and support respirations.
   b. Maintain warmth and prevent hypothermia.
   c. Ensure safety to prevent injury or infection.
   d. Identify actual or potential problems that might require immediate attention.

2. For continuing care
   a. Continue to protect from injury or infection and identify actual or potential problems that could require attention.
   b. Facilitate development of a close parent–infant relationship.
   c. Provide parents with information about newborn care.
   d. Assist parents in developing healthy attitudes about child-rearing practices.

C. Factors affecting newborn adaptation

1. Antepartal experiences of mother and newborn (e.g., exposure to toxic substances, parental attitude toward childbearing and childrearing)

2. Intrapartal experiences of mother and newborn (e.g., length of labor, type of intrapartal analgesia or anesthesia)

3. Newborn's physiologic capacity to make the transition to extrauterine life

4. Ability of health care providers to assess and respond appropriately in the event of potential problems

D. Nursing responsibilities

1. Support the neonate's physiologic adaptation to extrauterine life
2. Prevent or minimize potential complications
3. Facilitate parent–infant interaction

II. Transition to extrauterine life

A. Essential concepts

1. Immediate initiation of respiration and changes in the circulatory patterns are essential for extrauterine life.

2. Within 24 hours after birth, the newborn's renal, gastrointestinal (GI), hematologic, metabolic, and neurologic systems must function sufficiently for progression to and maintenance of extrauterine life.

B. **Transition period**

1. This is a phase of instability during the first 6 to 8 hours of life through which all newborns pass, regardless of gestational age or nature of labor and delivery.

2. In the first period of reactivity (immediately after birth), respiration is rapid (may reach 80 per minute) and transient nostril flaring, retractions, and grunting may occur. The heart rate may reach 180 beats per minute during the first few minutes of life.

3. Following this initial response, the newborn becomes quiet, relaxes, and falls asleep; this first sleep occurs within 2 hours of birth and lasts from a few minutes to several hours.

4. The second period of reactivity, starting when the newborn awakes, is marked by hyper-responsiveness to stimuli, skin color changes from pink to slightly cyanotic, and rapid heart rate.

5. Oral mucus may be a major problem during this period, causing choking, gagging, and coughing.

C. **Respiratory adaptation**

1. Initial respirations are triggered by physical, sensory, and chemical factors:

   a. Sensory factors: temperature, noise, light, sound, gravity; drop in temperature thought to be the most important

   b. Chemical factors: changes in the blood (decreased O_2 level, increased CO_2 level, decreased pH) as a result of the transitory asphyxia during delivery

   c. Physical factors: the effort required to expand the lungs and fill the collapsed alveoli; e.g., change in pressure gradients

2. Newborn respiratory rate ranges between 30 to 50 breaths per minute

3. Oral mucous secretions may cause the newborn to cough and gag, especially during first 12 to 18 hours.

4. Newborns are obligatory nose breathers: the reflex response to nasal obstruction is opening the mouth to maintain an airway; this response is not present in most newborns until 3 weeks after birth.

D. **Cardiovascular adaptation**

1. Various anatomical changes take place after birth, some immediate and others occurring over time (Table 11–1).

2. Peripheral circulation is sluggish, causing cyanosis of the hands and feet and around the mouth.

3. Pulse rate is 120 to 150 beats per minute while awake and 100 beats per minute while asleep.

4. Blood pressure averages 71/49 mmHg; varies with size and activity of newborn.

5. See Table 11–2 for normal newborn hematologic values

TABLE 11-1.
Changes in Fetal Circulation at Birth

STRUCTURE	BEFORE BIRTH	AFTER BIRTH
Umbilical vein	Brings arterial blood to liver and heart	Obliterated; becomes round ligament of liver
Umbilical arteries	Brings arteriovenous blood to placenta	Obliterated; become vesical ligaments on anterior abdominal wall
Ductus venosus	Shunts arterial blood into inferior vena cava	Obliterated; becomes ligamentum venosum
Ductus arteriosus	Shunts arterial and some venous blood from pulmonary artery to aorta	Obliterated; becomes ligamentum arteriosum
Foramen ovale	Connects right and left auricles (atria)	Obliterated usually; at times open
Lungs	Contains no air and very little blood	Filled with air and well supplied with blood
Pulmonary arteries	Brings little blood to lungs	Brings much blood to lungs
Aorta	Receives blood from both ventricles	Receives blood only from left ventricle
Inferior vena cava	Brings venous blood from body and arterial blood from placenta	Brings blood only to right auricle

Adapted from Guyton, A. C. (1986). *Medical physiology* (7th ed.). Philadelphia: W. B. Saunders.

TABLE 11-2.
Neonatal Blood Values

PARAMETER	NORMAL RANGE
Hemoglobin	15–20 g/dL
Red blood cells	5.0–7.5 million/mm^3
Hematocrit	43%–61%
White blood cells (WBCs)	10,000–30,000/mm^3
Neutrophils	40%–80%
Eosinophils	2%–3%
Lymphocytes	3%–10%
Monocytes	6%–10%
Immature WBC	3%–10%
Plateletes	100,000–280,000/mm^3
Reticlocytes	3%–6%
Blood volume	Early cord clamping: 78 mL/kg Late cord clamping: 98.6 mL/kg Third day after early cord clamping: 82.3 mL/kg Third day after late cord clamping: 92.6 mL/kg

E. **Temperature regulation and metabolic changes**

1. The newborn's temperature may drop several degrees after delivery, because the external environment is cooler than the intrauterine environment.
2. A limited supply of subcutaneous fat and a large skin surface area in relation to body weight predispose the newborn to heat transfer with the environment.
3. Rapid heat loss in a cool environment occurs by conduction, convection, radiation, and evaporation.
4. Cold stress (hypothermia) in the newborn, with its associated metabolic acidosis, can be lethal even for a vigorous, full-term newborn.

F. **Neurologic adaptation**

1. The newborn's neurologic system is not fully developed, either anatomically or physiologically.
2. The newborn exhibits uncoordinated movements; labile temperature regulation; poor control over musculature; easy startling, and tremors of the extremities.
3. Neonatal development is rapid, and the newborn soon develops more complex patterns of behavior (e.g., head control, smiling, and purposeful reaching)
4. Newborn reflexes are important indicators of the newborn's normal development (see Table 11–2)

G. **Gastrointestinal adaptation**

1. Enzymes for digestion are active at birth and can support extrauterine life by 36 to 38 weeks' gestation
2. The necessary muscular and reflex developments for transporting food are also present at birth.
3. Digestion of protein and carbohydrates is readily accomplished; fat digestion and absorption is poor due to the inadequacy of pancreatic enzymes and lipase.
4. Salivary glands are immature at birth, and little saliva is manufactured until age 3 months.
5. Meconium—greenish-black, viscous, and containing occult blood—is excreted within 24 hours in 90% of normal newborns.
6. Wide variations occur among newborns regarding interest in food, symptoms of hunger, and amount of food ingested at any one sitting.
7. Some newborns nurse immediately when put to the breast; others take up to 48 hours for effective feeding.
8. Random hand-to-mouth movement and sucking of fingers have been observed in utero; these actions are well developed at birth and are intensified with hunger.

H. **Kidney adaptation**

1. Glomerular filtration rate is relatively low at birth due to inadequate surface area of the glomerular capillaries.

2. Although these limitations do not compromise the healthy newborn, they do restrict the capacity of the newborn to respond to stressors.

3. Decreased ability to excrete drugs and excessive fluid loss can rapidly lead to acidosis and fluid imbalances.

4. Most newborns void in the first 24 hours after birth and 2 to 6 times per day for the first 1 to 2 days; thereafter, 5 to 20 times in 24 hours.

5. Urine may be cloudy due to mucus and urate; a reddish stain—"brick dust"—may be noticed on the diaper due to uric acid crystals.

I. Hepatic adaptation

1. During fetal life and to some degree after birth, the liver continues to aid in blood formation.

2. During the neonatal period, the liver produces substances essential for blood coagulation.

3. Iron stores from the mother are sufficient to carry the newborn through the fifth month of extrauterine life; at this time, the infant becomes susceptible to iron deficiency.

4. The liver also controls the amount of circulating unbound bilirubin, a pigment derived from the hemoglobin released with the breakdown of red blood cells.

5. Unconjugated bilirubin can leave the vascular system and permeate other extravascular tissues (e.g., the skin, sclera, oral mucous membranes), resulting in a yellow coloring termed jaundice.

6. In protracted cold stress, anaerobic glycolysis occurs, resulting in increased production of acids. Metabolic acidosis develops, and if there is a defect in respiratory function, respiratory acidosis also develops. Excessive fatty acids displace the bilirubin from the albumin-binding sites. The increased level of circulating unbound bilirubin that results increases the risk of kernicterus, even at serum bilirubin levels of 10 mg/dL or less.

J. Immune system adaptation

1. The newborn is unable to limit the invading organism at the portal of entry.

2. The immaturity of a number of protective systems significantly increases the risk of infection in the newborn period.

3. The inflammatory response is reduced both qualitatively and quantitatively.

4. Phagocytosis is sluggish.

5. The acidity of the stomach and the production of pepsin and trypsin, which maintain sterility of the small intestine, are not fully developed until 3 to 4 weeks of age.

6. IgA is missing from the respiratory and urinary tracts; unless the newborn is breast-fed, it is absent from the GI tract as well.

7. Infection represents one of the leading causes of morbidity and mortality during the neonatal period.

III. Essentials of newborn assessment

A. Neonatal health history

1. Comprehensive knowledge of the pregnancy, labor, and delivery is essential to understanding the significance of physical findings in the neonate.
2. A systematic approach helps ensure that pertinent data are not overlooked.
3. Major categories of data to obtain include:
   a. Maternal prenatal history and care
   b. Maternal blood type and Rh factor; history of isoimmunization, antibody titers
   c. Maternal screening tests results (e.g., rubella titer, hepatitis antigen screen, venereal disease research laboratory [VDRL], chlamydia screen, gonorrhea cultures, herpes cultures, human immunodeficiency virus screen)
   d. Labor history: onset, length, complication
   e. Rupture of membranes: amount of fluid, presence of meconium, relationship to time of delivery
   f. Fetal monitoring record (e.g., evidence of fetal distress, fetal scalp sampling, blood gas analysis results)
   g. Delivery history: length of second stage, medications and anesthesia (amount and when administered)
   h. Postnatal history (e.g., need for resuscitation, Apgars at 1 and 5 minutes)

B. Physical assessment

1. General appearance includes:
   a. Posture
   b. Skin color, wrinkling, vernix caseosa, milia, lanugo, erythema toxicum, birthmarks
   c. Respiratory effort
2. Vital sign and anthropometric assessment involves:
   a. Respiratory rate: counted for 60 seconds prior to determining apical rate while newborn is quiet; normal rate is 30 to 60 breaths per minute.
   b. Heart rate: apical rate counted for 60 seconds over the cardiac apex; normal rate is 120 to 160 beats per minute.
   c. Temperature: axillary temperature with thermometer held in axillary fold for 10 minutes; normal newborn temperature range is 36.4°C to 37.2°C (97.5°F to 99°F).
   d. Weight: weigh at the same time each day, prior to feeding; 95% of full-term newborns weight between 2500 g and 4250 g.
   e. Length: place on flat surface and extend legs fully before

measuring; average full-term length is 49.5 cm (19.5 inches).

 f. Head circumference: measure around the fullest part of the occiput; average head circumference is 35.5 cm.

 g. Chest circumference: place measure over the nipples and across the lower border of the scapulae; average circumference is 33 cm, usually 2 to 3 cm smaller than head.

 h. Blood pressure: not routinely measured at birth. Doppler ultrasound is the most accurate method in the neonate and provides systolic, diastolic, and mean arterial pressures; average blood pressure at birth is 80/46 mmHg

3. Detailed physical assessment involves:

 a. Head and face

  (1) Head size in proportion to body (normally about 25% of total body size)

  (2) Presence of molding

  (3) Symmetry of features

  (4) Ocular hypertelorism (wide-spaced eyes—a distance of more than 3 cm between inner canthi of the eyes)

 b. Fontanels

  (1) Anterior fontanel (normally diamond-shaped, 3 to 4 cm long and 2 to 3 cm wide; closes at 18 months)

  (2) Posterior fontanel (normally triangle-shaped, smaller than anterior; closes by 8 to 12 weeks)

  (3) Tense, bulging fontanel (may indicate increased intracranial pressure)

  (4) Sunken fontanel (characteristic of dehydration)

 c. Eyes

  (1) Color (usually appears blue or grey due to scleral thinness)

  (2) Transient strabismus and nystagmus (common)

  (3) Doll's eye phenomenon (may be seen when the head is turned and eye movements lag behind)

 d. Nose and mouth

  (1) Nasal patency, determined by closing the newborn's mouth and compressing one naris at a time

  (2) Mucous secretions (if excessive, may indicate tracheoesophageal fistula)

  (3) Precocious teeth, sucking calluses, and inclusion cysts (Epstein pearls)

 e. Ears and neck

  (1) Ear pliability and flexibility (in a full-term neonate, normally soft and pliable and recoil readily when bent forward)

        (2)   Low-set ears—top of ear below level of the eyes' canthi (may indicate a chromosomal or organ abnormality)

        (3)   Hearing (normally well developed once the eustachian tube is cleared)

        (4)   Neck size (normally short, with many thick folds)

        (5)   Neck webbing (associated with chromosomal abnormalities)

   f.   Chest

        (1)   Contour and symmetry (normally round and symmetrical)

        (2)   Breast engorgement (may be evident 2 to 3 days after birth due to maternal hormones)

        (3)   Respirations (normally shallow, symmetrical, and synchronous with abdominal movement)

        (4)   Breath sounds: rales (may be present during transitional period, representing fetal lung fluid and areas of atelectasis, and should clear within several hours); rhonchi (indicating fluid, mucus, or meconium in the larger bronchi and possibly associated with life-threatening conditions, such as meconium aspiration)

        (5)   Heart sounds (about 90% of all murmurs are transient and are related to incomplete closure of the foramen ovale or ductus arteriosus)

   g.   Abdomen

        (1)   Contour (normally rounded and protuberant due to weak abdominal musculature)

        (2)   Umbilical cord (normally appears white and gelatinous in the first few hours with two arteries and one vein apparent, and begins to dry within a few hours; shrunken, scaphoid appearance indicates diaphragmatic hernia)

        (3)   Bowel sounds (normally audible when newborn is relaxed)

   h.   Genitalia—female

        (1)   Labia minora (may have vernix and smegma in creases)

        (2)   Labia majora (normally cover the labia minora and clitoris)

        (3)   Clitoris (normally prominent)

        (4)   Vaginal discharge (may be present due to maternal hormones)

        (5)   Hymenal tag (normally present)

   i.   Genitalia—male

        (1)   Scrotum (normally rugae present on scrotum and both testes descended into scrotum)

                (2)   Penis (Urinary meatus normally located at tip of glans. Meatus on the dorsal surface is termed epispadias; on the ventral surface, hypospadias.)

    j.   Back and buttocks

          (1)   Spine (normally flat and round; tufts of hair or small indentations at the sacrum or base of the spine associated with spina bifida occulta)

          (2)   Patent anal opening

    k.   Upper extremities

          (1)   Flexion and movement (normally well flexed with symmetrical movement)

          (2)   Grasp reflex (normally present)

          (3)   Muscle tone and strength (partial or complete flaccidity of the arm may indicate trauma to brachial plexus)

          (4)   Brachial pulses (normally present)

    l.   Lower extremities

          (1)   Length and flexion (normally short, bowed, well flexed)

          (2)   Femoral and pedal pulses (normally present)

C. **Neurologic assessment (newborn reflexes)**

    1. Blink, cough, sneeze, and gag reflexes are present at birth and remain unchanged through adulthood.

    2. Several reflexes are normally present at birth, reflecting neurologic immaturity, and disappear in the first year. (See Table 11–3 for more information on neonatal reflexes.)

    3. Sensory behaviors

        a.   Vision:

          (1)   Can see objects at a distance of about 6 to 8 inches

          (2)   Prefers complex patterns to black and white

          (3)   Sensitive to light

          (4)   Can track parents with eyes

          (5)   Immature muscle coordination

        b.   Hearing: can detect sounds immediately

        c.   Taste

          (1)   Taste buds developed before birth

          (2)   Prefers sweet to bitter or sour tastes

        d.   Touch

          (1)   Can feel pressure, pain, and touch immediately or shortly after birth

          (2)   Sensitive to being cuddled

        e.   Smell

          (1)   After mucus and amniotic fluid cleared from nasal passages, can differentiate pleasant from unpleasant odors

TABLE 11–3.
Neonatal Reflexes

REFLEX	NORMAL RESPONSE	ABNORMAL RESPONSE
Rooting & sucking	Infant turns head in direction of stimulus, opens mouth, and begins to suck when cheek, lip or corner of mouth is touched with finger or nipple	Weak or absent response seen with prematurity, neurologic deficit or injury, or CNS depressions secondary to maternal drug ingestion (e.g., narcotics)
Swallowing	Infant swallows in coordination with sucking when fluid is placed on back of tongue	Gagging, coughing, or regurgitation of fluid; possibly associated with cyanosis secondary to prematurity, neurologic deficit, or injury; often seen after laryngoscopy
Extrusion	Infant pushes tongue outward when tip of tongue is touched with finger or nipple	Continuous extrusion of tongue or repetitive tongue thrusting seen with CNS anomalies and seizures
Moro	Bilateral symmetrical extension and abduction of all extremities, with thumb and forefinger forming characteristic "c," followed by adduction of extremities and return to relaxed flexion when infant's position is suddenly changed or if placed on back on flat surface	Asymmetrical response seen with peripheral nerve injury (brachial plexus) or fracture of clavicle or long bone of arm or leg No response with severe CNS injury
Stepping	Infant will step with one foot and then the other in walking motion when one foot is touched to flat surface	Asymmetrical response seen with CNS or peripheral nerve injury or fracture of long bone of leg
Prone crawl	Infant will attempt to crawl forward with both arms and legs when placed on abdomen on flat surface	Asymmetrical response seen with CNS or peripheral nerve injury or fracture of long bone
Tonic neck "fencing"	Extremities on side to which head is turned will extend and opposite extremities will flex when infant's head is turned to one side while resting. Response may be absent or incomplete immediately after birth	Persistent response after 4th month may indicate neurologic injury Persistent absence seen in CNS injury, neurological disorders
Startle	Infant abducts and flexes all extremities and may begin to cry when exposed to sudden movement or loud noise	Absence of response may indicate neurologic deficit or injury. Complete consistent absence of response to loud noises may indicate deafness. "Response may be absent or diminished during deep sleep.
Crossed extension	Infant's opposite leg will flex and then extend rapidly as if trying to deflect stimulus to other foot when placed in supine position and extending one leg while stimulating bottom of foot	Weak or absent response seen with peripheral nerve injury or fracture of long bone.
Glabellar "blink"	Infant will blink with first 4 or 5 taps to bridge of nose when eyes are open	Persistent blinking and failure to habituate suggestive of neurologic deficit

(continued)

TABLE 11–3.
Neonatal Reflexes (Continued)

REFLEX	NORMAL RESPONSE	ABNORMAL RESPONSE
Palmar grasp	Infant's finger will curl around object and hold momentarily when finger is placed in plam of infant's hand	Diminished response with prematurity Asymmetry with peripheral nerve damage (brachial plexus) or fracture of humerus No response with severe neurologic deficit
Planter grasp	Infant's toes will curl downward when a finger is placed against the base of the toes	Diminished response with prematurity No response with severe neurologic deficit
Babinski	Infant's toes will hyperextend and fan apart from dorsiflexion of big toe when one side of foot is stroked upward from heel and across ball of foot	No response with CNS deficit

Adapted from May, K. A., & Mahlmeister, L. R. (1990). *Comprehensive maternity nursing: Nursing process and the family* (2nd ed.) Philadelphia: J. B. Lippincott.

    (2)   Can distinguish mother's wet breast pad from other mothers' at 1 week

D. **Gestational age assessment**
1. Systematic assessment of physical signs and neurologic traits helps estimate the newborn's gestational age.
2. Degree of maturity at birth to a large extent determines the ability of the newborn to survive.
3. Determining gestational age provides information about system maturity and guides assessment for complications.

E. **Assessment of behavioral capabilities**
1. Individual personalities, behavioral characteristics and temperament play an important role in the ultimate relationship the newborn will form with parents and others.
2. By their actions, newborns encourage or discourage attachment and caretaking activities.
3. Awareness of the newborn's unique behavioral responses is important if parents are to learn to react to their newborn in ways that are health-promoting.
4. Brazelton and others have devised scales to evaluate newborn behavior.

IV. **Nursing management of the normal newborn: Transition period**

A. **Assessment**
1. Evaluate respiratory status; Apgar score at 1 and 5 minutes.
2. Assess general status: size (weight, length, head and chest circumference), gestational age, normality of body systems, vital signs.

    3. Measure axillary temperature every 30 minutes until stable, and every 4 hours thereafter.

    4. Assess blood sugar level on admission to the transition nursery and as indicated thereafter.

B. Nursing diagnoses

    1. Ineffective Airway Clearance

    2. Decreased Cardiac Output

    3. Altered Nutrition: Less than Body Requirements

    4. Ineffective Thermoregulation

C. Planning and implementation

    1. Maintain airway patency; assess frequently, keep a bulb syringe in bassinet.

    2. Maintain a neutral thermal environment by placing the newborn in radiant warmer; monitor temperature continuously using skin probe until stable. Delay bathing until temperature stabilizes; dry well after bath and return to radiant warmer until temperature is again stable.

    3. Protect from infection: observe aseptic technique and administer prophylactic ophthalmic antibiotics.

    4. Prevent nosocomial infection by instituting the following measures:

      a. Scrupulous handwashing technique

      b. "Clean" dress code (i.e., use of scrub attire on entering nursery and cover gowns as indicated)

      c. Pre-employment and annual staff physical examinations to identify organisms that might be transmitted to newborns

    5. Protect from hypoglycemia: observe for jitteriness, tremors, eye rolling, weakness, high-pitched cry, poor muscle tone; use Dextrostix, reporting to physician if less than 40 mg/dL; feed newborn according to established protocol (e.g., breast milk, glucose water, formula).

    6. Support establishment of feeding pattern.

    7. Support parent–newborn attachment.

    8. Prepare for routine procedures (e.g., identification of newborn, administration of vitamin K, and circumcision).

    9. Initiate a teaching plan, covering such issues as bathing, cord care, care of the uncircumcised male, circumcision care, diapering and dressing, dealing with crying, formula preparation and sterilization, feeding techniques, burping, elimination patterns, prevention and care of diaper rash, swaddling or wrapping, handling and carrying, temperature measurement, safety considerations, signs and symptoms of illness, administration of common medications (e.g., vitamins, antipyretics), clearing nasal passages with bulb syringe)

    10. If indicated, remind the parents when to return for outpatient laboratory studies (e.g., phenylketonuria, bilirubin).

D. **Evaluation**
1. The newborn breathes without assistance, as evidenced by normal respirations between 40 and 60 breaths per minute within 2 hours of birth.
2. The newborn maintains stable temperature, as evidenced by axillary temperature of 36.4°C to 37.2°C within 1 to 2 hours of birth.
3. The newborn demonstrates normal cardiac output, as evidenced by a regular heart rate of 120 to 160 beats per minute within 2 hours of birth.
4. The newborn shows no evidence of injury or infection.
5. The newborn begins to take nourishment within 4 to 8 hours of birth.
6. The mother demonstrates ability to feed the newborn by the time of discharge.
7. The newborn does not develop symptoms of hypoglycemia, or symptoms resolve without further complications with 12 to 24 hours.
8. The newborn and parents demonstrate interaction, as evidenced by touching, eye contact, and responsiveness to each other.

V. **Nursing management of the normal newborn: Continuing care**
A. **Assessment**
1. Continue assessing general status: size, maturation, normality of body systems, vital signs.
2. Evaluate fluid and caloric intake.
3. Assess elimination patterns.
4. Monitor and record weight gain or loss.

B. **Nursing diagnosis**
1. Constipation
2. Diarrhea
3. Fluid Volume Deficit
4. Altered Health Maintenance
5. Altered Nutrition: Less than Body Requirements
6. Altered Parenting

C. **Planning and implementation**
1. Promote adequate hydration and nutrition (newborn nutritional needs: calories, 120 cal/kg/day; fluid, 140 to 160 mL/kg/day).
2. Promote normal elimination patterns.
3. Promote positive parent–infant attachment.
4. Promote health maintenance (depending on the length of stay, discharge teaching is initiated on the unit and completed in the community during follow-up care of the family).
5. Recognize that discharge may occur as early as 6 hours after delivery, and plan teaching accordingly.

6. Arrange for ongoing assessment of newborn (and maternal) status (e.g., home follow-up visits and parent education classes).

D. Evaluation

1. The newborn regains birth weight by 7 to 14 days after birth.
2. The newborn demonstrates urinary and bowel elimination patterns within normal limits for mode of feeding.
3. Parents demonstrate growing comfort and ease in handling newborn by the time of discharge.
4. The newborn continues to make physiologic and behavioral adaptations and is screened for congenital conditions, as appropriate, within the first week of life.

Bibliography

Brunner, L. S., & Suddarth, D. S. (1987). *The Lippincott manual of nursing practice* (4th ed.). Philadelphia: J. B. Lippincott.

Danforth, D. N. (Ed.) (1986). *Obstetrics and gynecology* (5th ed.). Philadelphia: J. B. Lippincott.

Jensen, M. D., & Bobak, I. M. (1985). *Maternity and gynecologic care: The nurse and family* (3rd ed.). St. Louis: C. V. Mosby.

May, K. A., & Mahlmeister, L. R. (1990). *Comprehensive maternity nursing: Nursing process and the childbearing family* (2nd ed.). Philadelphia: J. B. Lippincott.

Olds, S. (1984). *Maternity-newborn nursing*. Menlo Park, CA: Addison-Wesley.

Reeder, S. J., & Martin, L. L. (1987). *Maternity nursing: Family, newborn, and women's health care* (16th ed.). Philadelphia: J. B. Lippincott.

Whaley, L. F., & Wong, D. L. (1987). *Nursing care of infants and children* (3rd ed.). St. Louis: C. V. Mosby.

STUDY QUESTIONS

1. The most effective means of preventing potential newborn for infection is which of the following?
   a. limitation of visitors
   b. wearing gown and gloves while caring for baby
   c. limit sibling visitation
   d. practicing good handwashing techniques

2. Vitamin K is given to the newborn soon after birth. The reason for this practice is which of the following?
   a. prevents jaundice in the newborn
   b. increases bilirubin breakdown
   c. aids in the clotting process
   d. aids in the development of antibodies

3. The nurse is observing the newborn's respiration to assess for the possibility of an ineffective breathing pattern. Which one of the following physiologic parameters would be the most important to know?
   a. Infants are able to breathe through both the nose and mouth.
   b. The respiratory rate should be 40 to 80 per minute.
   c. Newborn infants have slight sternal retraction with breathing, which is normal.
   d. Infants are obligatory nose breathers with respirations that are irregular and at a rate of 30 to 60 per minute.

4. Daily umbilical cord care to prevent the potential for infection should include which one of the following?
   a. Bathe daily with warm water and pat dry.
   b. Apply oil to the cord.
   c. Apply lotion to the area just next to the cord.
   d. Keep the cord and area directly surrounding clean and dry.

5. After circumcision of the male infant, which of the following is the most important nursing observation?
   a. The infant regains appetite.
   b. The infant has a normal stool.
   c. The infant voids normally.
   d. The infant does not develop a temperature.

6. When a nursing mother begins to breast-feed, the time allotted should be approximately which one of the following?
   a. 3 minutes per breast
   b. 10 minutes per breast
   c. 5 minutes per breast
   d. 15 minutes per breast

7. Which of the following positions for infant burping and actions by the person feeding the baby is the best?
   a. the baby lying on side and feeder stroking back
   b. the baby placed upright and feeder stroking back upward
   c. the baby placed upright and feeder stroking back downward
   d. the baby placed over shoulder

8. A nurse is conducting a postpartum parenting class. Which of the following maternal behavior would best satisfy the newborn infant's sensory need?
   a. stroking the infant's body
   b. rocking the infant
   c. singing to the infant
   d. stroking the infant's face

9. Newborns have the potential for infection. Which of the following is the most accurate reason for this occurence?
   a. They are exposed to so many health care workers.
   b. Rooming-in with family visitation can cause infection.
   c. The newborn has an immature immune system.
   d. The infant receives antibodies from the mother in pregnancy, so infection is not a problem.

10. You have completed a nursing assessment for gestational age and have found the following: sole creases over the anterior two thirds of the foot, 4 mm of breast tissue, fine fuzzy hair, and some

ear cartilage. You estimate this infant to be which of the following gestational ages?

a. 30 to 36 weeks
b. 36 to 38 weeks
c. 28 to 32 weeks
d. 41 to 42 weeks

ANSWER KEY

1. **Correct response: d**
   This is the best means of preventing infection.
   a. Visitors should wash hands and wear a gown, but limitation is not necessary.
   b. A gown is worn, but gloves are worn only before initial bath, if child is infected, and when inserting finger in mouth or anus.
   c. Limiting sibling visitation is rarely necessary.
   Application/Health promotion/ Implementation

2. **Correct response: c**
   Vitamin K aids in the clotting process.
   a. There is no medication to prevent jaundice.
   b. There is no medication to prevent bilirubin breakdown.
   d. There is no medication to aid in development of antibodies.
   Comprehension/Health promotion/ Implementation

3. **Correct response: d**
   Infants are obligatory nose-breathers; respirations are irregular and at a rate of 30 to 60 breaths per minute.
   a. Infants are not mouth-breathers.
   b. A rate above 60 breaths per minute indicate respiratory distress.
   c. Sternal retraction is an early sign of respiratory distress.
   Application/Physiologic integrity/Analysis

4. **Correct response: d**
   The cord and surrounding area should be kept clean and dry.
   a. The area should not be wet.
   b and c. Oil or lotion will clog pores and promote skin infection.
   Application/Health promotion/ Implementation

5. **Correct response: c**
   One wants to determine that the urethra was not damaged.
   a. Appetite will not be altered.

   b. Fecal elimination will not be altered.
   d. Circumcision is done under sterile conditions and should not cause infection.
   Application/Safe care/Evaluation

6. **Correct response: c**
   This time frame is a good middle ground.
   a. This is not quite enough time to stimulate milk production.
   b and d. This much stimulation initially could damage nipples.
   Application/Health promotion/ Implementation

7. **Correct response: b**
   Gentle stroking of the back upward will bring air upward.
   a. The baby should be upright.
   c. Placement is correct, but downward stroking will not bring air upward.
   d. Baby may eventually burp, but stroking will expedite the process.

8. **Correct response: a**
   Tactile stimulation of the whole body is necessary.
   b and c. These are not as important as tactile stimulation.
   d. Stroking the whole body is necessary.
   Application/Psychologic integrity/ Implementation

9. **Correct response: c**
   Immature immune system predisposes the newborn to infection.
   a. With proper infection control technique, this should not be a problem.
   b. Studies have shown the infection rate is not higher with rooming-in.
   d. The infant receives antibodies from the colostrum.
   Comprehension/Safe care/Analysis

10. **Correct response: b**
    Sole creases equal 38 weeks, breast tissue of 4 mm equals 38 weeks, fine fuzzy hair

equals 37 weeks, and ear cartilage equals 38 weeks.

 a and c. These characteristics would not be expected.

 d. Overdue babies have desquamating or peeling skin.

Comprehension/Physiologic integrity/Analysis

Antepartal Complications

I. Overview

A. Essential concepts

1. Although most pregnancies progress to successful delivery without complications, various factors can alter the physiologic processes of pregnancy and compromise the well-being of the mother or the developing fetus. These complications may occur at any time during pregnancy and can result from preexisting maternal medical problems or from the pregnancy itself.

2. Significant complications of pregnancy include:
   a. Hyperemesis gravidarum
   b. Anemia
   c. Hemolytic disease of the fetus or newborn
   d. Spontaneous abortion
   e. Placenta previa
   f. Abruptio placentae
   g. Ectopic pregnancy
   h. Pregnancy-induced hypertension (PIH)

3. Maternal conditions that can significantly affect the fetus or the progress of pregnancy include:
   a. Diabetes mellitus
   b. Cardiac disease
   c. Hematologic disorders (e.g., anemia, hemoglobinopathies)
   d. Infections
   e. Sexually transmitted diseases
   f. Substance abuse

4. Note that the disorders listed in Item 3 above are not covered in this chapter, because discussing all maternal conditions affecting pregnancy is beyond the scope of this book.

5. Major goals of prenatal nursing are screening for and preventing complications and developing therapeutic interventions.

6. Early and consistent prenatal care results in improved fetal and maternal outcome, regardless of complications that may occur.

B. General nursing management of at-risk antepartal patients

1. Assessment: Monitor each pregnancy to identify at-risk patients as early as possible.

2. Nursing diagnosis: in addition to the complication-specific diagnoses, the following nursing diagnoses are common to care of the at-risk antepartal patient:
   a. Anxiety
   b. Ineffective Family and Individual Coping
   c. Altered Family Processes
   d. Fear
   e. Altered Role Performance
   f. Self-concept Disturbance

g. Powerlessness

3. Planning and implementation: Initiate early intervention to prevent or alleviate problems.

4. Evaluation: The patient and family experience an optimal birth event, having coped successfully with a preexisting or emergent complication of pregnancy.

II. Hyperemesis gravidarum

A. Description: severe nausea and vomiting leading to electrolyte, metabolic, and nutritional imbalances in the absence of other medical problems

B. Etiology and pathophysiology

1. It is currently postulated that the rapidly increasing levels of human chorionic gonadotropin in early pregnancy induces emesis; however, this theory remains unproven.

2. Continued vomiting results in dehydration and ultimately decreases the amount of blood and nutrients circulated to the developing fetus.

3. Hospitalization may be required for severe symptoms when the patient needs intravenous hydration and correction of metabolic imbalances.

4. Signs and symptoms occur during the first 16 weeks of pregnancy and are intractable in nature.

C. Assessment findings

1. Signs and symptoms of hyperemesis gravidarum include:
   a. Unremitting nausea and vomiting
   b. Vomitus initially containing undigested food, bile, and mucus; later, blood and material resembling coffee grounds
   c. Weight loss

2. Associated findings may include:
   a. Pale, dry skin
   b. Subnormal or elevated temperature
   c. Rapid pulse
   d. Fetid, fruity breath odor from acidosis
   e. Central nervous system effects such as confusion, delirium, headache, and lethargy, stupor, or coma

D. Nursing diagnoses

1. Anxiety
2. Fluid Volume Deficit
3. Altered Nutrition: Less than Body Requirements

E. Planning and implementation

1. Administer intravenous fluids as ordered; may be done on a outpatient basis when dehydration is mild.

2. Monitor and record intake and output.

3. Maintain a nonjudgmental atmosphere in which the patient and family can express concerns and resolve some of their fears.

F. **Evaluation**
1.   The patient responds to treatment; nausea and vomiting subside, weight gain is maintained.
2.   The patient keeps follow-up appointments to assess progress of pregnancy.

III. **Anemia**

A. **Description: hemoglobin value of 10 g or less during the second and third trimesters**

B. **Etiology and pathophysiology**
1.   Causes of anemia include nutritional deficiency (iron deficiency, megaloblastic anemia—which includes both folic acid deficiency and B_{12} deficiency), acute and chronic blood loss, and hemolysis (sickle cell anemia, thalassemia, G6PD)
2.   Iron deficiency anemia is common during pregnancy, affecting 15% to 50% of pregnant women
3.   Mild anemia (Hg 11 g) poses no threat but is seen as an indication of a less than optimal nutritional state
4.   Maternal morbidity is uncommon unless hemoglobin level drops below 6 g
5.   More subtle complications—delayed wound healing, infection, postpartum hemorrhage—are associated with less severe reductions in hemoglobin level
6.   Hemoglobinopathies such as thalassemia, sickle cell disease, and G6PD lead to anemia by causing hemolysis or increased destruction of red blood cells

C. **Assessment findings**
1.   A pregnant woman with hemoglobin level below 10.5 g may complain of excessive fatigue, headache, and tachycardia.
2.   Severe iron deficiency anemia may cause brittle fingernails, cheilosis, or a smooth, red, shiny tongue.

D. **Nursing diagnoses**
1.   Ineffective Individual and Family Coping
2.   Knowledge Deficit
3.   Altered Nutrition: Less than Body Requirements

E. **Planning and implementation**
1.   Provide teaching about iron supplementation and dietary sources of iron, as indicated.
2.   Teach aspects of self-care and symptoms of complications.
3.   Prepare for type and cross-match for packed cells during labor in the presence of severe anemia.
4.   In a pregnant patient with thalassemia, provide support, particularly if she is just becoming aware that she is carrying the trait; carefully assess for signs of infection during the pregnancy.
5.   In a pregnant patient with sickle cell disease, assess iron and

folate stores and reticulocyte counts; complete screening for hemolysis; provide dietary counseling and folic acid supplements; monitor for infection.

6. In a pregnant patient with G6PD, provide iron and folic acid supplementation and nutrition counseling, and teach the patient to avoid oxidizing drugs.

F. Evaluation

1. The patient and family verbalize understanding of anemia.
2. The patient complies with the treatment regimen.
3. The patient maintains adequate nutrition.
4. Hemoglobin levels respond to treatment, and pregnancy continues without related untoward events.

IV. Hemolytic disease of fetus and newborn

A. Description: an immune reaction by the mother's blood against the blood group factor on the fetus's red blood cells

B. Etiology and pathophysiology

1. This disorder occurs when the fetus inherits a blood group antigen from the father that the mother does not possess. The mother's body forms an antibody against that particular blood group antigen, and hemolysis begins.
2. It may result from ABO or Rh incompatibility.
3. ABO incompatibility occurs in about 20% of pregnancies.
4. Rh incompatibility occurred in about 1.5% of all pregnancies before prophylactic RhoGAM (Rh immune globulin) became available in the mid-1960s; incidence is much lower now.

C. Assessment findings

1. The hemolytic response in ABO incompatibility is usually mild, and phototherapy usually can resolve the resulting newborn jaundice.
2. In the Rh-negative mother, Rh incompatibility leads to varying degrees of anemia and jaundice (erythroblastosis fetalis) if the fetus is Rh-positive.

D. Nursing diagnoses

1. Anxiety
2. Knowledge Deficit
3. Fear

E. Planning and Implementation

1. Provide appropriate and accurate information relative to the treatment and care anticipated
2. Expect to administer RhoGAM at 28 weeks' gestation even when titers are negative. (note: this is recommended practice by the ACOG to protect against the effects of early transplacental hemorrhage.)
3. Ensure that the mother is cross-matched with RhoGAM; coor-

dination with the laboratory for the injection "set-up" is necessary.

4. Focus management of the immunized Rh-negative mother on close monitoring of fetal well-being, as reflected by Rh titers, amniocentesis results, and sonography.

5. When the Rh-negative mother is in labor, cross-match for Rho-GAM to be given within 72 hours of delivery.

6. If the mother becomes sensitized, and there is evidence of erythroblastosis, notify the perinatal team of the possibility for delivery of a compromised infant.

F. Evaluation

1. The patient responds to treatment; antibody titers remain within normal limits.

2. The patient continues follow-up appointments to assess progress of pregnancy.

V. Spontaneous abortion

A. Description

1. Spontaneous abortion is defined as premature expulsion from the uterus of the fetus or other products of conception.

2. Spontaneous abortion may be classified as:

   a. Threatened: cramping and vaginal bleeding in early pregnancy with no cervical dilation; may subside or follow with an incomplete abortion

   b. Imminent or inevitable: bleeding, cramping, and cervical dilation; termination cannot be prevented

   c. Incomplete: expulsion of only part of the products of conception (placenta); bleeding with cervical dilation

   d. Complete: complete expulsion of all products of conception

   e. Missed: early fetal intrauterine death and products of conception are not expelled; cervix closed, there may be a dark brown vaginal discharge, negative pregnancy test, and cessation of uterine growth and breast tenderness

   f. Habitual: spontaneous abortion of three or more consecutive pregnancies

B. Etiology and pathophysiology

1. Spontaneous abortion may result from fetal, placental, or maternal factors.

2. Fetal factors include:

   a. Defective embryologic development

   b. Faulty ovum implantation

   c. Rejection of the ovum by the endometrium

3. Placental factors include:

   a. Premature separation of the normally implanted placenta

      b.   Abnormal placental implantation
      c.   Abnormal platelet function
   4. Maternal factors include:
      a.   Infection
      b.   Severe malnutrition
      c.   Reproductive system abnormalities (e.g., incompetent cervix)
      d.   Endocrine problems (e.g., thyroid dysfunction)
      e.   Trauma
      f.   Drug ingestion

C. **Assessment findings**
   1. Common signs and symptoms of spontaneous abortion include:
      a.   Vaginal bleeding in the first 20 weeks of pregnancy
      b.   Complaints of cramping in lower abdomen
      c.   Fever, malaise, or other symptoms of infection
      d.   Dry skin or mucous membranes, thirst, nausea, anorexia
   2. The patient and family may also exhibit behaviors suggestive of normal or morbid grief reaction at the loss of pregnancy, such as:
      a.   Crying
      b.   Depression
      c.   Sustained or prolonged social isolation
      d.   Withdrawal

D. **Nursing diagnoses**
   1. Fluid Volume Deficit
   2. Anticipatory Grieving
   3. Dysfunctional Grieving
   4. High Risk for Infection

E. **Planning and implementation**
   1. Monitor vital signs, bleeding, and cramping or pain.
   2. Assess history of previous pregnancies.
   3. Offer emotional support and anticipatory guidance relative to expected recovery, need for rest, and delaying another pregnancy until the patient is fully recovered.
   4. Suggest avoiding intercourse until after the next menses or using condoms when engaging in intercourse.
   5. Recommend iron supplements and increase in dietary iron as indicated.
   6. Prepare for RhoGAM administration to a Rh-negative mother, as ordered.
   7. Monitor intravenous fluids, vital signs, and laboratory studies in the presence of heavy vaginal bleeding; prepare for surgery if indicated.
   8. Provide emotional support because the couple may experience

blame, guilt, grief, and loss; teach about the condition and aspects of self-care.

F.   **Evaluation**

1.   The patient responds to teaching about diet, iron supplementation, and rest.
2.   The patient and family demonstrate behaviors associated with normal grieving without signs of morbid grief reaction.
3.   The patient remains free of infection.
4.   The patient responds to iron supplementation by maintaining normal blood values.
5.   The patient maintains fluid volume balance, as evidenced by normal vital signs and hydration status.

VI.   **Placenta previa**

A.   **Description**

1.   In this disorder, the placenta implants in the lower uterine segment, causing painless bleeding in the second and sometimes third trimester of pregnancy.
2.   Placenta previa may be classified as:
     a.   Total: placenta completely covers the internal os
     b.   Partial: placenta partially covers the internal os
     c.   Low lying or low implantation: placenta reaches to the area of the internal os

B.   **Etiology and Pathophysiology**

1.   Pathologic process seems to be related to the conditions that alter the normal function of the uterine decidua and its vascularization.
2.   Predisposing factors include:
     a.   Multiparity (80% of affected patients are multiparous)
     b.   Advanced maternal age (older than 35 accounts for 33% of cases)
     c.   Multiple gestation
     d.   Previous cesarean birth
     e.   Uterine incisions
     f.   Prior placenta previa (incidence is 12 times greater in women who have had a previous previa)
3.   Bleeding results from tearing of the placental villi from the uterine wall as the lower uterine segment contracts and dilates; can be slight or profuse.
4.   Incidence is one in 300 deliveries.

C.   **Assessment findings**

1.   Signs and symptoms of placenta previa include:
     a.   Bright red, painless bleeding
     b.   Abdomen soft, nontender, and relaxes between contractions
     c.   Fetal outline palpable

      d.   Fetal heart rate (FHR) stable within normal limits
      e.   Fetal presenting part unengaged
   2.   Diagnosis can be made by ultrasound (indirect) or by feeling the placenta through the cervical os (direct). Caution must be used with pelvic examination, because it can cause further tearing of villi and profuse bleeding.

D. **Nursing diagnoses**
   1.   Activity Intolerance
   2.   Fear
   3.   Dysfunctional Grieving
   4.   High Risk for Infection
   5.   Sleep Pattern Disturbance

E. **Planning and implementation**
   1.   Monitor vital signs and bleeding
   2.   Observe for shock (rapid pulse, pallor, cold moist skin, fall in blood pressure)
   3.   Monitor FHR
   4.   Provide strict bed rest to minimize the risk to the fetus.
   5.   Observe for further bleeding episodes; prepare for ambulation and discharge, which may be within 48 hours of last bleeding episode.
   6.   Provide emotional support during the grieving process.
   7.   Provide patient teaching about the condition and expected management: cover the need to have immediate transportation to the hospital available at all times, to come to the hospital at once if further bleeding occurs, and to avoid intercourse until after delivery.

F. **Evaluation**
   1.   The patient demonstrates increasing activity tolerance.
   2.   The patient and family exhibit functional grieving.
   3.   The patient remains free from infection.
   4.   The patient gets adequate sleep and rest, reports feeling.

VII. Abruptio placenta
A. **Description: premature separation of a normally implanted placenta during the second half of pregnancy, often with severe hemorrhage**
B. **Etiology and pathophysiology**
   1.   The cause of abruptio placentae is unknown.
   2.   Risk factors include:
      a.   Uterine anomalies
      b.   Multiparity
      c.   PIH
      d.   Previous cesarean delivery
      e.   Renal or vascular disease
      f.   Trauma to abdomen

        g.   Previous third trimester bleeding

        h.   Abnormally large placenta

    3.   If the patient is in active labor and bleeding cannot be stopped via bed rest and tocolytics, emergency cesarean delivery may be indicated.

C.   **Assessment findings**

    1.   Signs and symptoms of abruptio placenta include:

        a.   Concealed or external dark red bleeding

        b.   Uterus firm to board-like, with severe continuous pain

        c.   Uterine outline possibly enlarged or changing shape

        d.   FHR present or absent

        e.   Fetal presenting part may be engaged

    2.   Severe abruptio placentae may produce such complications as:

        a.   Severe hemorrhage and shock

        b.   Renal failure

        c.   Disseminated intravascular coagulation

        d.   Maternal and fetal death

D.   **Nursing diagnoses**

    1.   Fear

    2.   High Risk for Fluid Volume Deficit

    2.   Knowledge Deficit

    3.   Pain

E.   **Planning and implementation**

    1.   Continuously evaluate maternal and fetal physiologic status, including:

        a.   Vital signs

        b.   Bleeding

        c.   Electronic fetal and maternal monitoring

        d.   Signs of shock—rapid pulse, pallor, cold and moist skin, fall in blood pressure

    2.   Never perform a vaginal or rectal examination or take any action that would stimulate uterine activity.

    3.   Provide emotional support and teach about the condition.

    4.   Assess the need for immediate delivery.

F.   **Evaluation**

    1.   The patient remains free of complications.

    2.   Pregnancy progresses to delivery without further incident.

VIII.   **Ectopic pregnancy**

    A.   **Description: implantation of products of conception in a site other than endometrium (e.g., fallopian tube, ovary, cervix, peritoneal cavity)**

    B.   **Etiology and pathophysiology**

        1.   Ectopic pregnancy can result from conditions that hinder ovum passage through the fallopian tube and into the uterine cavity, such as:

        a.   Endosalpingitis
        b.   Diverticula
        c.   Tumors
        d.   Adhesions from previous surgery
        e.   Transmigration of the ovum from one ovary to the opposite fallopian tube

    2.   Maternal prognosis is good with early diagnosis and prompt treatment; rarely, the fetus survives to term in cases of abdominal implantation.

C. **Assessment findings**
    1.   Ectopic pregnancy sometimes produces signs and symptoms of normal pregnancy or may be asymptomatic.
    2.   Common clinical manifestations include:
        a.   Dizziness, syncope
        b.   Sharp abdominal pain, referred shoulder pain
        c.   Vaginal bleeding
        d.   Adnexal mass and tenderness
    3.   Rupture of a fallopian tube can produce life-threatening complications, such as hemorrhage, shock, and peritonitis

D. **Nursing diagnosis**
    1.   Anxiety
    2.   Dysfunctional Grieving
    3.   Knowledge Deficit
    4.   Pain

E. **Planning and implementation**
    1.   Monitor vital signs, bleeding, and pain.
    2.   Teach about the condition and aspects of self-care.
    3.   Provide emotional support as the patient grieves for her lost pregnancy.

F. **Evaluation**
    1.   The patient remains free of complications.
    2.   The patient verbalizes understanding of the condition.
    3.   The patient exhibits functional grieving.

IX. **PIH**

A. **Description**
    1.   PIH is a hypertensive disorder of pregnancy developing after 20 weeks' gestation and characterized by edema, hypertension, and proteinuria.
    2.   PIH can take two forms: preeclampsia and eclampsia.

B. **Etiology and pathophysiology**
    1.   The cause of PIH is unknown.
    2.   Possible contributing factors include:
        a.   Poor prenatal care, particularly inadequate nutrition
        b.   Primigravid status
        c.   Multiple pregnancy

        d.   Preexisting maternal diabetes mellitus or hypertension

        e.   Infection

        f.   Exposure to toxins

C. **Assessment findings**

  1. Manifestations of mild preeclampsia include:

      a.   Increase in systolic blood pressure 30 mmHg or increase in diastolic blood pressure 15 mmHg above baseline, noted on two readings taken 6 hours apart

      b.   Generalized edema in face, hands, and ankles

      c.   Weight gain of 1.5 kg/month in second trimester or greater that 0.5 kg/week in third trimester

      d.   Proteinuria 1+ to 2+

  2. Severe preeclampsia is marked by:

      a.   Blood pressure >160/110 mmHg noted on two readings taken 6 hours apart with the patient on bed rest

      b.   Proteinuria >5 g/24 hours

      c.   Oliguria (<400 mL/24 hours)

      d.   Headache

      e.   Blurred vision, spots before eyes, retinal edema

      f.   Pitting edema of legs

      g.   Dyspnea

      h.   Epigastric pain

      i.   Nausea and vomiting

      j.   Hyperreflexia

      k.   Anxiety, irritability.

  3. Eclampsia may produce:

      a.   Blood pressure >160/110 mmHg

      b.   Grand mal seizures

      c.   Coma

D. **Nursing diagnoses**

  1. Anxiety

  2. High Risk for Injury

  3. Knowledge Deficit

  4. Pain

E. **Planning and implementation**

  1. Monitor vital signs, FHR.

  2. Minimize external stimuli, promote rest and relaxation.

  3. Monitor urine output, protein, and specific gravity.

  4. Assess for edema of face, arms, hands, legs, ankles, and feet, and for pulmonary edema.

  5. Check weight daily.

  6. Assess deep tendon reflexes every 4 hours.

  7. Assess for placental separation, headache and visual disturbance, epigastric pain, and altered level of consciousness.

  8. Provide treatment as ordered, which may include:

      a.   For mild preeclampsia: bed rest in left lateral recumbent position; balanced diet with moderate to high protein and low to moderate sodium

      b.   For severe preeclampsia: complete bed rest; balanced diet with high protein and low to moderate sodium; anticonvulsants; magnesium sulfate; fluid and electrolyte replacements; sedative (Valium or phenobarbital); antihypertensives

      c.   For eclampsia: magnesium sulfate intravenously

   9.   Institute seizure precautions

  10.   Provide emotional support and teaching about condition

F.   **Evaluation**

   1.   The patient remains free of serious complications, or exhibits resolution of complications.

   2.   The patient verbalizes understanding of the disorder and treatment measures.

   3.   Pregnancy progresses to term without major incident.

Bibliography

Brunner, L. S., & Suddarth, D. S. (1987). *The Lippincott manual of nursing practice* (4th ed.). Philadelphia: J. B. Lippincott.

Danforth, D. N. (Ed.) (1986). *Obstetrics and gynecology* (5th ed.). Philadelphia: J. B. Lippincott.

Jensen, M. D., & Bobak, I. M. (1985). *Maternity and gynecologic care: The nurse and family* (3rd ed.). St. Louis: C. V. Mosby.

May, K. A., & Mahlmeister, L. R. (1990). *Comprehensive maternity nursing: Nursing process and the childbearing family* (2nd ed.). Philadelphia: J. B. Lippincott.

Olds, S. (1984). *Maternity-newborn nursing.* Menlo Park, CA: Addison-Wesley.

Reeder, S. J., & Martin, L. L. (1987). *Maternity nursing: Family, newborn, and women's health care* (16th ed.). Philadelphia: J. B. Lippincott.

STUDY QUESTIONS

1. Tracy King, a 35-year-old gravida II, para 0, comes to the clinic after her second spontaneous abortion. She asks the nurse, "Why am I having miscarriages?" The nurse's best response would be that each case is different, but most spontaneous abortions are linked to
   a. fetal defects incompatible with life
   b. advanced maternal age
   c. inadequate maternal nutrition
   d. placental abnormalities

2. Rose Royce, a 29-year-old gravida III para II at 23 weeks' gestation, is admitted to the labor and delivery unit with painless, bright red vaginal bleeding. Rose reports that she has been feeling tired and has noticed ankle swelling in the evening. Laboratory tests reveal a hemoglobin level of 11.5 g/dL. After evaluating the situation, the nurse determines that Rose is at risk for placenta previa, based on which of the following data?
   a. anemia
   b. edema
   c. painless vaginal bleeding
   d. fatigue

3. When caring for a patient with a possible diagnosis of placenta previa, which of the following admission procedures should the nurse omit?
   a. perineal shave
   b. enema
   c. urine specimen collection
   d. blood specimen collection

4. Which of the following is a classic symptom of pregnancy-induced hypertension (PIH)?
   a. edema of the feet and ankles
   b. edema of the hands and face
   c. weight gain of 1 lb/week
   d. early morning headache

5. Mary MacKay came to the clinic in the last week before her estimated date of confinement complaining of headaches, blurred vision, and vomiting. Suspecting advanced PIH, the nurse would best respond to Mary's complaints with which of the following statements?
   a. "The doctor probably will want to admit you for observation."
   b. "The doctor probably will order bed rest at home."
   c. "These are really dangerous signs."
   d. "The doctor will prescribe some medicine for you."

6. Which of the following blood pressure parameters indicates PIH? Elevation over baseline of
   a. 30 mmHg systolic and/or 15 mmHg diastolic
   b. 40 mmHg systolic and/or 20 mmHg diastolic
   c. 10 mmHg systolic and/or 5 mmHg diastolic
   d. 20 mmHg systolic and/or 20 mmHg diastolic

7. When discussing possible complications of pregnancy with a patient, the nurse would explain that all of the following are symptoms of urinary tract infection during pregnancy *except*
   a. low back pain
   b. urinary frequency
   c. GI distress
   d. malaise

8. The nurse should prepare a pregnant woman with active genital herpes for which of the following types of delivery?
   a. induction
   b. mid forceps rotation
   c. low forceps
   d. cesarean

ANSWER KEY

1. *Correct response: a*
   Fetal abnormality is the leading cause of spontaneous abortion.
   b, c, and d. Although advanced maternal age, poor maternal nutrition, and placental defects are all possible causes of spontaneous abortion, fetal abnormality is the leading cause.
   Comprehension/Physiologic/Implementation

2. *Correct response: c*
   In placenta previa, changes in the lower uterine segment during the later months of pregnancy cause placental separation from the attachment site, marked by vaginal bleeding.
   a. Rose's hemoglobin level is within the normal range during pregnancy.
   b. Ankle edema is a normal physiologic phenomenon of pregnancy, resulting from pressure by the enlarged uterus on great vessels and lymphatics.
   d. Fatigue is common during pregnancy.
   Application/Physiologic/Analysis (Dx)

3. *Correct response: b*
   An enema could dislodge the placenta and increase bleeding.
   a. Perineal shave would not aggravate the condition.
   c and d. Laboratory data are important in planning care.
   Comprehension/Safe care/Implementation

4. *Correct response: b*
   Edema of the hands and face is a classic sign of PIH
   a. Many healthy pregnant women experience foot and ankle edema.

   c. Weight gain of 2 lb or more per week is indicative of a problem.
   d. Early morning headache is not a classic sign of PIH.
   Knowledge/Safe care/Assessment

5. *Correct response: b*
   The patient with advanced PIH needs rest, and home usually is the best place to get it.
   a. Hospitalization probably would not be necessary in this situation.
   c. This response is not professional and could cause increased anxiety in the patient.
   d. Medication is not indicated in this situation.
   Analysis/Safe care/Analysis (Dx)

6. *Correct response: a*
   These are accepted parameters for mild PIH.
   b, c, and d. These parameters are incorrect.
   Knowledge/Physiologic/Assessment

7. *Correct response: b*
   Frequency commonly occurs during pregnancy, and thus is not necessarily a sign of UTI.
   a, c, and d. These are all symptoms of urinary tract infection.
   Comprehension/Physiologic/Implementation

8. *Correct response: d*
   Cesarean delivery will help prevent transmission of infection to the newborn during vaginal delivery.
   a, b, and c. Vaginal delivery can transmit herpes infection to the newborn.
   Application/Safe care/Implementation

Intrapartal Complications

I. Overview

A. Essential concepts

1. Problems that can be anticipated because of maternal or fetal conditions or that can be stabilized and corrected without emergency intervention are increasingly managed in facilities designed to accommodate high-risk maternal and fetal patients.

2. In situations where the expectant mother is the best "incubator" for the high-risk neonate, she may be transported to a tertiary care facility.

3. Because intrapartal emergencies commonly develop rapidly, on-the-spot nursing assessment and intervention is crucial.

4. Principles of nursing care during normal labor (see Chapter 9, Intrapartal Care) apply to complicated labor as well.

B. General nursing management of at-risk intrapartal patients

1. Assessment
   a. Determine the presence of predisposing factors.
   b. Provide intensive monitoring and support of maternal and physiologic status, with emphasis on early detection of changes and efficient implementation of appropriate interventions.
   c. Evaluate the family's responses to labor and to the crisis situation.

2. Nursing diagnoses: in addition to complication-specific diagnoses, the following nursing diagnoses are common to care of the at-risk intrapartal patient:
   a. Anxiety
   b. Altered Cardiac Output
   c. Ineffective Individual and Family Coping
   d. Anticipatory Grieving: Dysfunctional
   e. High Risk for Injury
   f. Knowledge Deficit
   g. Fear
   h. Pain
   i. Self-concept Disturbance
   j. Spiritual Distress
   k. Altered Tissue Perfusion
   l. Altered Patterns of Urinary Elimination

3. Planning and implementation
   a. Monitor and support maternal and fetal physiologic status.
   b. Provide anticipatory guidance for the patient and her partner.
   c. Coordinate patient care efforts (typically, patients with intrapartal complications require intravenous fluids and

a variety of medical procedures and treatments such as electronic monitoring, central venous lines, medications, and retention catheters).

    d.   Expect the unexpected and be prepared to provide critical care nursing if needed.

    4.   Evaluation

        a.   The patient and fetus maintain normal physiologic status; any deviations that arise are identified and corrected early.

        b.   The patient and partner understand procedures to be performed as indicated by their questions and their restatement of information provided to them.

        c.   The couple experiences decreased fear and anxiety and increased comfort, as evidenced by verbal expressions of appreciation for support and increased use of coping techniques.

II. Induction of labor

  A. **Overview**

    1.   The deliberate initiation of labor prior to the start of spontaneous contractions may be either mechanical (amniotomy or rupture of amniotic membranes), physiologic (ambulation, maternal position change, nipple stimulation), or chemical (prostaglandins and oxytocin).

    2.   Artificial rupture of membranes (AROM) may be adequate stimulation to initiate contractions; AROM may be done after oxytocin stimulation has established effective contractions.

    3.   AROM is initiated when the cervix is soft, partially effaced, and slightly dilated—preferably when the fetal presenting part is engaged.

    4.   Oxytocin induction must be done with careful, ongoing monitoring; oxytocin is a very powerful drug. Hyperstimulation of the uterus may result in tetanic contractions prolonged to over 70 seconds, which could cause such complications as fetal distress due to impaired uteroplacental perfusion, abruptio placentae, amniotic fluid embolism, laceration of the cervix and uterine rupture, and neonatal trauma.

  B. **Nursing implications: AROM**

    1.   Explain the procedure and inform the patient that labor usually follows within 6 to 8 hours of AROM and that contractions can be expected to be more intense and to expect leakage of fluid.

    2.   Monitor fetal heart tones immediately prior to, during, and after the procedure.

    3.   Observe and record color, amount, and odor of fluid, time of procedure, and cervical status.

172

    4.   Monitor the patient's temperature every 2 hours to assess for infection.

C.   Nursing management: Oxytocin induction

    1.   Review the hospital's policy relative to the amount, rate, and interval of use of oxytocin.

    2.   Use infusion pump for precise regulation of the medication.

    3.   Observe for signs of hypertonicity, such as contractions >75 mmHg, >90 seconds duration, or closer than 2 minutes, and be prepared to immediately discontinue the oxytocin.

    4.   Initiate continuous internal or external fetal monitoring and evaluate for normal range of 120 to 160 beats per minute. If there is loss of variability, late decelerations, or persistent bradycardia (<120 beats per minute), discontinue oxytocin infusion, administer O_2, notify physician, reposition patient to left side or opposite side, initiate internal fetal monitoring, and perform a vaginal examination—fetal distress may be result of rapid labor progress, descent of fetus, or cord prolapse.

    5.   Monitor and record vital signs and fetal heart rate (FHR) every 15 to 30 minutes; assess for signs of impending delivery

III. Cesarean delivery

A.   Overview

    1.   In this surgical procedure, the infant is delivered through an incision made through the maternal abdomen

    2.   Previously called a C-section; the preferred term is now cesarean birth or cesarean delivery.

    3.   Currently, the U.S. incidence of cesarean birth ranges between 15% and 20%; up from 4% in the mid-1960s.

    4.   It may be planned (elective) or arise from an unanticipated problem (emergency).

    5.   Types of cesarean delivery include:

        a.   Classic: a vertical midline skin incision is made in the skin and the body of the uterus; permits easier access to the fetus and thus is indicated in emergency situations, when there are abdominal adhesions from previous surgeries, or when the fetus is in a transverse lie; blood loss is increased because large blood vessels of the myometrium are involved; because the uterine musculature is weakened, there is greater possibility of rupture of the uterine scar in subsequent pregnancies.

        b.   Low segment: in this, the most common type, the skin incision is low ("bikini" or Pfannenstiel incision) and the uterine incision is horizontal in the lower uterine segment; blood loss is minimal, fewer postdelivery complications occur, and the incision is easy to repair, with less chance of rupture of uterine scar during future deliveries; the procedure takes longer to perform than the classic incision; it is therefore not useful in emergencies.

6. A trial of labor and vaginal birth after cesarean is increasingly regarded as a safe and appropriate mode of obstetric management.

7. Elective, repeat cesarean may be performed in the absence of a specific indication for operative delivery when either the physician or the patient is unwilling to attempt vaginal delivery.

8. Anesthesia may be either general or spinal; preoperative and postoperative care will vary accordingly.

B. Assessment

1. Obtain a complete obstetric history.
2. Assess condition and signs of labor.
3. Determine frequency, duration, and intensity of contractions.
4. Determine condition of fetus through fetal heart tones (FHTs), fetal monitoring strips, fetal scalp blood sample, fetal activity changes, presence of meconium in amniotic fluid.
5. Observe the patient and family for emotional response and ability to cope with discomfort and pain

C. Nursing diagnoses

1. Anxiety
2. Body Image Disturbance
3. Ineffective Family and Individual Coping
4. Fear
5. High Risk for Fluid Volume Deficit
6. High Risk for Injury
7. Knowledge Deficit
8. Pain
9. Altered Patterns of Urinary Elimination

D. Implementation

1. Modify preoperative teaching to meet the needs of planned versus emergency cesarean birth; depth and breadth of instruction will depend on the circumstances and time available.

2. Facilitate a family-centered cesarean birth by including, when possible, such activities as:
   a. Prepare the partner for participation in the delivery.
   b. Reunite the family as soon as possible following delivery.
   c. Provide for family time alone in the critical first hours after the mother and baby are stabilized.
   d. Include the father (and siblings, when possible) in teaching of care-giving skills.

3. Provide preoperative preparation for major abdominal surgery (i.e., shave and antiseptic skin preparation, insert urinary catheter, obtain preoperative laboratory tests, insert intravenous line, obtain informed consent, ensure correct patient identifi-

cation, notify other health team members that delivery is imminent).

4. Provide intraoperative care for both mother and baby (i.e., timing and documenting of events, immediate care of the newborn).

5. Provide immediate postoperative care following cesarean birth, which is similar to care of a patient after vaginal birth plus care of the postabdominal surgery patient (i.e., meeting physiologic and psychosocial needs after delivery, after surgery, and after anesthesia).

6. If the newborn is compromised, provide additional support and attention as indicated.

7. If the parents give evidence of feelings of failure as new parents because a "normal" birth experience wasn't achieved, provide additional time to relive and talk through the experience with reassuring support.

8. Refer for home care and follow-up visit, as indicated by mother's and infant's status and length of hospital stay.

9. Assist family in planning for care of mother and infant at home, taking into consideration need for increased rest (influenced by type of anesthesia, length of labor, type of abdominal or uterine incision), inability to climb stairs, drive car.

E. Evaluation

1. The patient progresses toward recovery without postsurgical or postbirth complications, as evidenced by appropriate vital signs, and contracted uterus and appropriate amount of lochia in first 5 days after birth.

2. The patient recovering from cesarean birth responds to analgesia and is comfortable, as evidenced by verbalization of comfort, more relaxed countenance, relaxation in holding newborn, and stabilizing vital signs.

3. The patient maintains appropriate intake and output and ability to void within 12 hours of delivery.

4. The patient progresses toward recovery without complications, as evidenced by normal vital signs, appropriate wound healing, and normal lochia.

5. The couple demonstrate beginning of attachment and parenting, as evidenced by interest in reviewing cesarean birth with nurse, discussing care procedures, and participating in return demonstrations in care of the newborn.

IV. **Preterm labor**

A. **Description:** labor that begins after 20 weeks' gestation and before 37 weeks' gestation

B. **Etiology and pathophysiology**

1. Among the many causes of preterm labor are:

      a.   Premature rupture of the membranes (PROM)

      b.   Preeclampsia

      c.   Hydramnios

      d.   Placenta previa

      e.   Abruptio placentae

      f.   Incompetent cervix

      g.   Trauma

      h.   Uterine structural anomalies

      i.   Congenital adrenal hyperplasia

      j.   Fetal death

   2.   Maternal risk factors include age under 18 years, history of preterm labors, multiple pregnancy, hydramnios, smoking, poor hygiene, poor nutrition, employment.

C.   Assessment findings

   1.   Manifestations of preterm labor are the same as those of labor at term, including:

      a.   Rhythmic uterine contractions

      b.   Cervical dilatation and effacement

      c.   Possible rupture of membranes

      d.   Expulsion of the cervical mucous plug

      e.   Bloody show

   2.   Obstetric history reveals gestation not to term.

D.   Nursing diagnoses

   1.   Anxiety

   2.   Fear

   3.   High Risk for Injury

   4.   Knowledge Deficit

E.   Planning and implementation

   1.   Obtain a thorough obstetrical history

   2.   Assess condition and signs of labor

   3.   Determine frequency, duration, and intensity of uterine contractions

   4.   Determine cervical dilatation and effacement

   5.   Assess status of membranes and presence of "bloody show."

   6.   Evaluate fetus for fetal distress, size, maturity (sonography and lecithin–sphingomyelin ratio).

   7.   Test vaginal discharge for amniotic fluid with Nitrazine paper.

   8.   Relieve anxiety by providing information of status and support.

   9.   Provide comfort measures and adequate hydration.

   10.   Encourage bed rest in side-lying position.

   11.   Administer oxygen, 8 to 12 L/min by mask.

   12.   Facilitate laboratory tests: complete blood count, urinalysis.

   13.   Prepare for possibility of ultrasound, amniocentesis, tocolytic drug therapy, steroid therapy.

      14. Administer tocolytic medications as ordered.

      15. Assess for side effects of tocolytic therapy (e.g., decreased maternal blood pressure, dyspnea, chest pain, and FHR >180 beats per minute).

  F. **Evaluation**

      1. The patient responds to treatment by cessation of preterm labor.

      2. Fetus responds to treatment, as evidenced by normal monitoring results and pregnancy continues.

      3. The patient verbalizes her fears; cooperates with staff.

      4. The patient and family verbalize understanding of medical procedures and expected neonatal outcome.

      5. The patient copes with decreased mobility and verbalizes understanding of the rationale for limiting activity.

V. PROM

  A. **Description: rupture of the chorion and amnion 1 hour or more before the onset of labor**

  B. **Etiology and pathophysiology**

      1. The precise cause and specific predisposing factors are unknown.

      2. PROM is known to be associated with malpresentation, possible weak areas in the amnion and chorion, subclinical infection and, possibly, incompetent cervix.

      3. Amniotic fluid leaks from the vagina in the absence of contraction.

      4. Increased risk of ascending intrauterine infection is known as chorioamnionitis.

      5. Basic and effective defense against fetus contracting infection is lost; the leading cause of death associated with PROM is infection.

      6. When the latent period (time between rupture of membranes and onset of labor) is short—less than 24 hours—the risk of infection is low.

      7. Management is affected by the gestational age of the fetus and estimates of viability.

  C. **Assessment findings**

      1. PROM is marked by blood-tinged amniotic fluid gushing from the vagina.

      2. Maternal fever, fetal tachycardia, and malodorous discharge point to infection.

  D. **Nursing diagnoses**

      1. Anxiety

      2. Fear

      3. High Risk for Infection

      4. High Risk for Injury

      5. Knowledge Deficit

E. Planning and implementation

    1. Determine maternal and fetal status, including estimated gestational age.

    2. Make an early and accurate evaluation of membrane status using sterile speculum examination and Nitrazine paper testing; thereafter, keep vaginal examinations to a minimum.

    3. Obtain smear specimens from vagina and rectum, as ordered, to test for beta-hemolytic streptococci, an organism that increases the risk to the fetus.

    4. In the presence of evidence to suggest leaking amniotic fluid, periodic assessment for early signs of infection are indicated.

    5. Inform the patient, if the fetus is at term, that the chances of spontaneous labor beginning are excellent; encourage the patient and partner to prepare themselves for labor and birth.

    6. Should labor not begin or the fetus is judged to be preterm or at high risk for infection, explain treatments that are likely to be needed.

    7. Maintain patient on bed rest if fetal head engaged in order to prevent cord prolapse should additional rupture and loss of fluid occur.

F. Evaluation

    1. The patient and family verbalize accurately understanding of the situation and cooperate with care.

    2. The patient and fetus experience no further complications and delivery progresses.

VI. Dystocia

A. Description: difficult, painful, prolonged labor due to mechanical factors

B. Etiology

    1. Fetal factors (passenger): unusually large fetus, fetal anomaly, malpresentation and malposition

    2. Uterine factors (powers): hypotonic labor, hypertonic labor, precipitous labor, prolonged labor

    3. Pelvic factors (passage): inlet contracture, midpelvis contracture, outlet contracture

    4. "Psyche" factors: maternal anxiety and fear, or lack of preparation

C. Assessment findings

    1. Dystocia is marked by decreased strength of uterine contractions and decreased uterine tone after the onset of true labor.

    2. Contractions may become farther apart and irregular.

D. Nursing diagnoses

    1. Anxiety

    2. Fear

3. High Risk for Fluid Volume Deficit
4. High Risk for Infection
5. High Risk for Injury
6. Knowledge Deficit
7. Pain

E. Planning and implementation

1. Assess uterine contractions for dysfunctional patterns by both palpation and electronic monitor.
2. Assess condition of fetus by monitoring FHR, fetal activity, and color of amniotic fluid.
3. Check patient's level of fatigue and ability to cope with pain.
4. Assess maternal vital signs: temperature, pulse, respiration, and blood pressure.
5. Check maternal urine for acetone (an indication of dehydration and exhaustion).
6. Provide emotional support by explaining progress and procedures and giving encouragement and appropriate reassurance.
7. Provide comfort by promoting relaxation through bathing and keeping the patient and bed clean, back rubs, frequent position changes (sidelying); encourage walking if indicated, quiet environment.
8. Encourage human support and contact; coach in breathing and relaxation techniques.
9. Encourage frequent emptying of bladder; catheterize as indicated.

F. Evaluation

1. The patient avoids exhaustion.
2. The patient achieves as much comfort as possible.
3. The patient avoids panic and discouragement.
4. The patient avoids bladder distention.
5. The patient retains normal fluid volume.
6. The patient is free of infection.

VII. Uterine rupture

A. Description: abrupt tearing of the uterus, either complete (rupture extends through entire uterine wall and the uterine contents are spilled into the abdominal cavity) or incomplete (rupture extends through the endometrium and myometrium, but the peritoneum surrounding the uterus remains intact)

B. Etiology and pathophysiology

1. Most common predisposing factor is a preexisting scar that results in a weakened or defective myometrium that does not stretch; most frequently indicated in spontaneous uterine rupture.
2. Traumatic uterine rupture may be caused by trauma from obstetrical instruments, such as uterine sound or curette or tools

used in abortion, or from obstetric intervention, such as excessive fundal pressure, forceps delivery, violent bearing-down efforts, tumultuous labor, shoulder dystocia.

3. Spontaneous uterine rupture is most likely to occur following previous uterine surgery, grand multiparity combined with the use of oxytocic agents, cephalopelvic disproportion, mal presentation, or hydrocephalus.

4. More severe ruptures pose the risk of irreversible maternal hypovolemic shock or subsequent peritonitis and the consequent fetal anoxia, and fetal or neonatal death.

5. Small tears may be asymptomatic and may heal spontaneously, remaining undetected until the stress and strain of a subsequent labor.

6. If signs of possible uterine rupture are present, vaginal delivery is generally not attempted.

7. If symptoms are not severe, an emergency cesarean delivery may be attempted with repair of the uterine tear.

8. If symptoms are severe, emergency laparotomy will be performed to attempt immediate delivery of the fetus and then establish homeostasis.

C. **Assessment findings**
   1. Signs and symptoms vary from very mild to very severe, depending on the site and extent of the rupture, degree of extrusion of the uterine contents, and the occurrence or absence of intraperitoneal spill of amniotic fluid and blood.
   2. Common findings include:
      a. Abdominal pain
      b. Vaginal bleeding
      c. Lack of progress in labor
   3. In complete uterine rupture, the mother may exhibit signs of hypovolemic shock

D. **Nursing diagnoses**
   1. Anxiety
   2. Fear
   3. Fluid Volume Deficit
   4. High Risk for Injury
   5. Knowledge Deficit
   6. Pain

E. **Planning and implementation**
   1. In the presence of predisposing factors, monitor maternal labor pattern closely for hypertonicity or signs of weakening uterine muscle
   2. Recognize signs of impending rupture and immediately notify the physician and call for assistance.
   3. Take the steps in *ORDER* to prevent or limit hypovolemic

shock: *O*, oxygenate (8 to 10 L/min using closed mask); *R*, restore circulating volume (one or more IV lines); *D*, drug therapy (be prepared to digitalize, have emergency drugs readily available); *E*, evaluate (cause, response to therapy, fetal condition); and *R*, remedy the problem (surgery, antibiotics).

4. Implement the following preparations for surgery:
   a. Monitor maternal blood pressure, pulse and respirations, and FHTs.
   b. Establish a CVP catheter to permit assessment of blood loss and monitor effects of fluid and blood replacement.
   c. Insert a urinary catheter for precise determinations of fluid balance.
   d. Obtain blood for assessment of acidosis.
   e. Administer oxygen and maintain a patent airway.

5. Provide support for partner and family members once surgery has begun; inform them how they will receive information about the mother and baby.

F. Evaluation

1. Signs of uterine rupture are recognized immediately; appropriate and timely interventions follow.

2. The patient and fetus respond to therapeutic interventions without sequelae.

VIII. Uterine inversion

A. **Description: the uterus turns completely or partially inside out; occurs immediately following delivery of the placenta or in the immediate postpartum period.**

B. **Etiology and pathophysiology**

1. Forced inversion caused by excessive pulling of the cord or vigorous manual expression of the placenta or clots from an atonic uterus.

2. Spontaneous inversion due to increased abdominal pressure because of bearing down, coughing, or sudden abdominal muscle contraction.

3. Predisposing factors include straining after delivery of placenta, vigorous kneading of the fundus to expel the placenta, manual separation and extraction of the placenta, rapid delivery with multiple gestation, or rapid release of excessive amniotic fluid

4. Immediate manual replacement of the uterus at the time in inversion will prevent cervical entrapment of the uterus; if reinversion is not performed immediately, rapid and extreme blood loss may occur, resulting in hypovolemic shock.

C. **Assessment findings**

1. In the unanesthetized patient, excruciating pelvic pain in conjunction with a sensation of extreme fullness extending in to the vagina heralds inversion.

  2. Once inversion occurs, the patient may exhibit a dramatic increase in vaginal bleeding, accompanied by increasing pulse rate or other signs of hemorrhage.

D. **Nursing diagnoses**
  1. Fear
  2. Fluid Volume Deficit
  3. High Risk for Injury
  4. Pain

E. **Planning and implementation**
  1. Recognize signs of impending inversion and immediately notify the physician and call for assistance
  2. Take the steps in *ORDER* to prevent or limit hypovolemic shock (see section VIII.E.3).
  3. If manual reinversion is not successful, prepare the patient and family for possibility of general anesthesia and surgery

F. **Evaluation**
  1. Signs of uterine inversion are recognized immediately; appropriate and timely interventions follow.
  2. The patient and infant respond to therapeutic interventions without sequelae.

IX. **Cord prolapse**

A. **Description: descent of the umbilical cord into the vagina before the fetal presenting part and compression of the cord between the presenting part and the maternal pelvis, compromising or completely cutting off fetoplacental perfusion**

B. **Etiology and pathophysiology**
  1. Occurs most frequently with prematurity, unengaged cephalic presentations with ruptured membranes, shoulder or footling breech presentations
  2. May follow rupture of amniotic membranes because the fluid rush may carry the cord along toward the birth canal
  3. Occurs in one out of 200 pregnancies
  4. Cord prolapse is an emergency situation; immediate delivery will be attempted to save the fetus.
  5. When delivery is accomplished within 15 to 30 minutes, fetal survival is 70% to 75%; fetal mortality may exceed 50% if delivery is delayed more than 1 hour.

C. **Assessment findings**
  1. The prolapsed cord may be visible or palpable.
  2. Signs of acute fetal distress may develop as the cord is compressed.

D. **Nursing Diagnoses**
  1. Anxiety
  2. Fear
  3. High Risk for Injury

E. Planning and implementation

1. Assess a laboring patient often if fetus is preterm or small for gestational age, if fetus has not engaged, or if the patient has PROM.
2. Periodically evaluate FHR, especially immediately following rupture of membranes (spontaneous or surgical), and again in 5 to 10 minutes.
3. Lower head of bed and elevate maternal hips on pillow or place patient in knee-chest position to minimize pressure on the cord.
4. Apply firm manual pressure to the presenting part of the fetus upward with sterile gloved hand to elevate it and relieve pressure from the cord.
5. Assess cord pulsations constantly.
6. Notify physician and prepare for cesarean birth.
7. Provide information and support to woman and family.

F. Evaluation

1. The patient and family verbalize understanding of the situation and cooperate with care.
2. The patient and fetus experience no further complications and delivery progresses.
3. The patient and family verbalize a decreased level of anxiety.

X. Early postpartum hemorrhage

A. Description: blood loss of 500 mL or more during the first 24 hours after delivery (see Chapter 14 for discussion of hemorrhage that occurs later in the postpartum period)

B. Etiology and pathophysiology

1. Postpartum hemorrhage is the leading cause of maternal death worldwide; more common cause of excessive blood loss during early postpartum period.
2. Approximately 5% of women experience some type of postdelivery hemorrhage.
3. Major causes of postpartum hemorrhage are uterine atony (responsible for at least 80% of all early postpartum hemorrhages); laceration of cervix, vagina, or perineum; and retained placental fragments.
4. Predisposing factors include hypotonic contractions, overdistended uterus, multiparity, large infant, forceps delivery, and cesarean delivery.

C. Assessment findings

1. Vaginal bleeding is the obvious sign of postpartal hemorrhage; amount and character vary with cause.
2. Excessive blood loss may produce hypotension, thready pulse, pallor, restlessness, dyspnea, and chills.

D. Nursing diagnoses
1. Anxiety
2. Body Image Disturbance
3. Decreased Cardiac Output
4. Ineffective Individual and Family Coping
5. Fluid Volume Deficit
6. Impaired Gas Exchange
7. High Risk for Injury
8. Knowledge Deficit
9. Pain
10. Powerlessness
11. Altered Tissue perfusion: Cardiopulmonary

E. Planning and implementation
1. Determine presence of uterine atony through frequent periodic assessment of uterine firmness and amount of vaginal bleeding immediately after delivery.
2. Monitor serial maternal vital signs postdelivery—every 5 to 15 minutes until stable, increasing or decreasing frequency relative to baseline and amount of bleeding.
3. Provide gentle fundal massage, taking care to support the uterus with the hand just above the symphysis pubis.
4. Administer intravenous oxytocin as ordered.
5. Keep an accurate pad count (100 mL per saturated pad).
6. Monitor condition of skin, urinary output, and level of consciousness.
7. Allay anxiety through explanation and reassurance.

F. Evaluation
1. The patient's condition stabilizes and she progresses through normal involution stages.
2. Parent–infant contact is supported and maintained as the mother's physiologic condition stabilizes.

Bibliography

Brunner, L. S., & Suddarth, D. S. (1987). *The Lippincott manual of nursing practice* (4th ed.). Philadelphia: J. B. Lippincott.

Danforth, D. N. (Ed.) (1986). *Obstetrics and gynecology* (5th ed.). Philadelphia: J. B. Lippincott.

Jensen, M. D., & Bobak, I. M. (1985). *Maternity and gynecologic care: The nurse and family* (3rd ed.). St. Louis: C. V. Mosby.

May, K. A., & Mahlmeister, L. R. (1990). *Comprehensive maternity nursing: Nursing process and the childbearing family* (2nd ed.). Philadelphia: J. B. Lippincott.

Olds, S. (1984). *Maternity-newborn nursing*. Menlo Park, CA: Addison-Wesley.

Reeder, S. J., & Martin, L. L. (1987). *Maternity nursing: Family, newborn, and women's health care* (16th ed.). Philadelphia: J. B. Lippincott.

STUDY QUESTIONS

1. When assessing a patient whose membranes have ruptured, the nurse notes that the fluid is a greenish color. What is the cause of this greenish coloration?
   a. blood
   b. meconium
   c. hydramnios
   d. caput

2. With a breech presentation, the nurse must be particularly alert for which of the following?
   a. quickening
   b. ophthalmia neonatorum
   c. pica
   d. prolapsed umbilical cord

3. Following the rupture of membranes, fetal distress in a vertex presentation may be indicated by which of the following?
   a. bloody show
   b. hydramnios
   c. oligohydramnios
   d. meconium

4. Based on the preceding question, which of the following nursing interventions should receive the highest priority?
   a. Assess FHR.
   b. Call the physician.
   c. Assess maternal vital signs.
   d. Assess maternal emotional status.

5. Joan, age 26 years, has begun spotting during the third trimester. It has been determined that it is too early to initiate labor. Joan is therefore placed on bed rest at home. Her forced immobility has placed extra strain on her marital relationship and on family relationships in general. Her husband is protective one moment and angry at her helplessness the next. She feels guilty and angry about the disruption in the healthy pregnancy and in her family life. Based on this information, the nurse would most likely deem which of the following nursing diagnoses as the most important to the family at this time?
   a. Fear related to uncertainty of the future
   b. Knowledge deficit related to disrupted (crisis) pregnancy
   c. High Risk for Dehydration related to hemorrhage
   d. Ineffective family coping related to disrupted (crisis) pregnancy

6. Which of the following nursing interventions would *not* be appropriate for a patient just admitted with vaginal bleeding in the third trimester of pregnancy?
   a. careful admission history
   b. specific assessment of amount of bleeding
   c. vaginal examination to determine progress of cervical dilation
   d. vital signs every 15 minutes

7. Mrs. Adams is brought into the emergency room following a car accident. She is in her third trimester of pregnancy and states that she was wearing her seatbelt. She has no external evidence of injury, but complains of severe abdominal pain. Her abdomen is enlarging and is rigid upon palpation. Fetal monitoring indicates acute fetal distress. Mrs. Adams is likely experiencing which of the following complications?
   a. placenta previa
   b. abruptio placentae
   c. severe abdominal bruising
   d. normal labor stimulated by stress

8. The prognosis for fetal survival following abruptio placentae is less than 50%. For infants who survive, there is a high degree of morbidity. Knowing this, nursing intervention should focus on which of the following?
   a. monitoring maternal physiologic status
   b. monitoring maternal and infant physiologic status
   c. providing emotional support regarding the imminent delivery of a deceased or defective baby
   d. administering tocolytic agents to arrest labor

9. Mrs. Allen, who is at term in her pregnancy, arrives at the hospital stating that her "waters broke" an hour ago, but she

has not begun labor. The nurse's analysis of this information would lead to which of the following conclusions?

a. The patient is at high risk for chori-amnionitis.
b. Cesarean delivery is likely.
c. The risk of infection is low at present.
d. Fetal distress or death is likely.

ANSWER KEY

1. **Correct response: b**
   Upon descent into the pelvis, the fetus in a breech presentation will pass meconium due to compression on the intestinal tract.
   a. Greenish amniotic fluid is not an indication of bleeding.
   c. Hydramnios refers to an excessive amount of amniotic fluid.
   d. Caput is the occiput of the fetal head that appears at the vaginal introitus just before delivery of the head.
   Analysis/Safe care/Analysis (Dx)

2. **Correct response: d**
   There is space available between the presenting part and the cervix, through which the cord can slip.
   a. Quickening is the woman's first perception of fetal movements.
   b. Conjunctivitis of the newborn is generally due to maternal gonorrhea.
   c. Pica refers to the abnormal oral intake of substances such as cornstarch, dirt, clay, or plaster by a malnourished individual, often by a child or pregnant woman in need of nutrients to support growth.
   Analysis/Safe care/Analysis (Dx)

3. **Correct response: d**
   With fetal distress there is an increase in the peristaltic movement of the intestines; thus the fetus will expel meconium.
   a. Bloody show is the pink mucus discharge that is present after discharge of the mucous plug. Show is caused by pressure from the fetal presenting part upon the cervix, causing rupture of capillaries.
   b. Hydramnios refers to an excessive amount of amniotic fluid.
   c. Oligohydramnios refers to a decreased amount of amniotic fluid, frequently seen with a fetal urinary tract anomaly.
   Application/Safe care/Assessment

4. **Correct response: a**
   Meconium-stained amniotic fluid is a sign

of fetal distress and the FHR must be assessed immediately.
   b, c, and d. Although these are important areas to assess, none is the highest priority given the risk to the fetus.
   Evaluation/Health promotion/Planning

5. **Correct response: d**
   In this situation, Ineffective Family Coping would be the priority diagnosis.
   a, b, and c. The other responses could be possible nursing diagnoses, but the data support ineffective coping as the priority family concern or issue.
   Application/Psychosocial/Analysis (Dx)

6. **Correct response: c**
   Vaginal examination should not be performed or damage to fetal blood vessels may occur and hemorrhage might worsen.
   a, b, and d. These are all appropriate nursing interventions in this situation.
   Knowledge/Safe care/Implementation

7. **Correct response: b**
   The assessment data are typical of abruptio placenta.
   a, c, and d. The data do not support any of the other disorders listed.
   Application/Physiologic/Analysis (Dx)

8. **Correct response: b**
   Both mother and infant should be monitored carefully to promote survival and to decrease risk of morbidity.
   a. The infant must be monitored as well as the mother.
   c. Fetal death or defects may not occur.
   d. Tocolytics are contraindicated in abruptio placentae.
   Application/Safe care/Implementation

9. **Correct response: c**
   When the latent period is less than 24 hours, the risk of infection is low.

a. The risk for chorioamnionitis would be low in this patient.
b. Spontaneous labor within 24 to 48 hours is likely in term mothers, thereby obviating the need for cesarean delivery.
d. Term infants are at lowest risk for distress or death.

Analysis/Safe care/Analysis (Dx)

Postpartal Complications

I.   Overview

A.   Essential concepts

1. Today, relatively short postpartal hospitalizations (for most pa-
    tients, 24 to 72 hours) require that the nurse focus postpartal

care on assisting parents to care for themselves and their infant effectively.

2. Preexisting maternal health problems (e.g., anemia, pregnancy-induced hypertension, diabetes) contribute to many postpartal complications.

3. Overall nursing objectives for high-risk postpartal patients include:

   a. Provide prompt diagnosis and treatment of postpartal complications to minimize risk of morbidity, mortality, and dysfunctional effects.

   b. Promote comfort and recovery through physical care measures, nutrition, and pain-relief therapies.

   c. Provide patient and family teaching to improve their understanding and integration of the experience.

   d. Minimize separation of mother and infant and assist in developing the mother–infant relationship through information, support, and encouragement of mother–infant attachment.

   e. Assist the patient and family to deal with anxiety, anger, grief, and fear through self-expression and acceptance.

B. General nursing management for high-risk postpartal patients

1. Assessment: monitor the following:

   a. Vital signs
   b. Patterns of temperature elevation
   c. Condition of perineum and uterus
   d. Character of lochia
   e. Tenderness and pain
   f. Condition of legs
   g. Condition of breasts
   h. Status of bladder and voiding
   i. Rest and sleep
   j. Appetite, nutrition, and hydration
   k. Pain or discomfort
   l. Relation to infant
   m. Response to complication
   n. Response to partner

2. Nursing diagnoses: in addition to complication-specific diagnoses, the following nursing diagnoses are common to at-risk postpartal patients:

   a. Anxiety
   b. Ineffective Individual and Family Coping
   c. Altered Family Processes
   d. Fear
   e. Knowledge Deficit
   f. Pain
   g. Altered Parenting

3. Planning and implementation
    a. Record and report signs and symptoms.
    b. Administer medications and treatments.
    c. Monitor vital signs.
    d. Collect specimens.
    e. Monitor fluids and hydration status.
    f. Provide physical care.
    g. Enhance fluid and food intake.
    h. Carry out treatment regimen (e.g., sitz baths, medications, dressings).
    i. Encourage maximum mother–infant contact; provide continuous information on the infant.
    j. Explain and discuss complication, expected course and treatment.
    k. Involve partner in education about complication, infant, mother's need for emotional support.
4. Evaluation
    a. The mother's vital signs are stabilized.
    b. The mother voids completely.
    c. The mother remains symptom free.
    d. The mother rests and sleeps well.
    e. The mother takes adequate fluids and food.
    f. The mother reports relief from pain and discomfort.
    g. The mother assumes as much caretaking of infant as her condition permits.
    h. The mother maintains interest in infant.
    i. The mother and family understand treatment and expected course of complication.
    j. The mother and family express grief and fear.

II. Postpartum hemorrhage and subinvolution
A. Description
1. Postpartum hemorrhage: blood loss of more than 500 mL following birth
2. Subinvolution: delayed involution of puerperal structures
B. Etiology and pathophysiology
1. Early postpartum hemorrhage occurs in first 24 hours after delivery, usually due to uterine atony, lacerations, or retained placental fragments (see Chapter 13, Intrapartal Complications, for information on nursing care related to early postpartum hemorrhage).
2. Late postpartum hemorrhage occurs after the first 24 hours after delivery, generally caused by retained placental fragments or bleeding disorders.
3. Subinvolution results from retained placental fragments and membranes, endometritis, or uterine fibroid; treatment depends on cause.

C. **Assessment findings**
1. Vaginal bleeding is the obvious sign of postpartal hemorrhage; amount and character vary with cause.
2. Signs of impending shock include changes in skin temperature and color and altered level of consciousness.

D. **Nursing diagnoses**
1. Anxiety
2. Fear
3. Fluid Volume Deficit
4. High Risk for Infection
5. High Risk for Injury
6. Knowledge Deficit
7. Pain

E. **Planning and implementation**
1. Massage uterus, facilitate voiding, report blood loss.
2. Prepare for intravenous infusion, oxytocin, and blood transfusions, if needed.
3. Administer medications and oxygen, as ordered.
4. Monitor blood pressure, pulse every 5 to 15 minutes.
5. Monitor intake and output.
6. Support and communicate with the patient and family members during an emergency situation, thus enhancing cooperation with resuscitative efforts.
7. Teach self-care techniques as appropriate (e.g., fundal massage, assessing fundal height and consistency, and inspecting episiotomy and lacerations)
8. Teach importance of rest and adequate nutrition

F. **Evaluation**
1. The mother returns to stable condition and normal involution.
2. The mother can verbalize stages of normal involution, knows danger signs.
3. The mother knows how to assess for abnormal bleeding.
4. The mother demonstrates ability to manage self-care.

III. **Puerperal infection**

A. **Description: infection developing in the birth structures after delivery**

B. **Etiology and pathophysiology**
1. Puerperal infection is a major cause of maternal morbidity and mortality. Incidence ranges from 1% to 8% of all deliveries; higher incidence in cesarean deliveries.
2. Major site of postpartum infections is the pelvic cavity; other common sites include the breasts, urinary tract, and venous system.
3. Puerperal morbidity is marked by temperature elevation of

38°C (100.4°F) or higher after the first 24 hours postpartum on any two of the first 10 postpartum days.
4. Causative organisms include the following:
   a. Aerobic: beta-hemolytic streptococci, *Escherichia coli*, *Klebsiella*, *Proteus mirabilia*, Pseudomonas, *Staphylococcus aureus*, and Neisseria
   b. Anaerobic: bacteroides, peptostreptococcus, peptococcus, and *Clostridium perfringens*
5. Localized infections include lesions of vagina, vulva, and perineum.
6. Endometritis, localized infection of the uterine lining, occurs 48 to 72 hours after delivery.
7. In parametritis (pelvic cellulitis), infection spreads by way of lymphatics of connective tissue surrounding the uterus.
8. Puerperal infection may be extended to the peritoneum by way of the lymph nodes and wall of the uterus.

C. **Assessment findings**
   1. Localized vaginal, vulval, and perineal infections are marked by pain, elevated temperature, edematous, reddened, firm and tender at site of wound; sensation of heat; burning on urination; and discharge from wound.
   2. Manifestations of endometritis include rise in temperature for several days, if severe: malaise, headache, backache, general discomfort, loss of appetite; large tender uterus, severe postpartum cramping, brownish-red foul lochia.
   3. Parametritis (pelvic cellulitis) commonly produces elevated temperature (102°F to 104°F), chills, abdominal pain, subinvolution of uterus, tachycardia, and lethargy.
   4. Signs and symptoms of peritonitis include high fever, rapid pulse, abdominal pains, nausea, vomiting, and restlessness

D. **Nursing diagnoses**
   1. High Risk for Injury
   2. Knowledge Deficit
   3. Pain

E. **Planning and implementation**
   1. Inspect perineum twice daily for redness, edema, ecchymosis, and discharge.
   2. Evaluate for abdominal pain, fever, malaise, tachycardia, foul-smelling lochia.
   3. Obtain specimens, report findings.
   4. Encourage balanced diet, frequent fluids, and early ambulation.
   5. Administer antibiotics or medications, noting response.
   6. Teach self-care, stressing careful perineal hygiene, handwashing.

F. **Evaluation**
1. The mother remains pain free.
2. The mother performs self-care.
3. The mother verbalizes accurate understanding of her condition.

IV. Mastitis
A. **Description: inflammation of the breast tissue or abscess formation in glandular tissue**
B. **Etiology and pathophysiology**
1. Injury to breast is the primary predisposing factor (e.g., over-distention, stasis, cracking of nipples).
2. Probable sources of infection:
    a. Epidemic infection: derived from nosocomial source, usually *Staphylococcus aureus*; localizes in the lactiferous glands and ducts
    b. Endemic infection: occurs randomly and localizes in the periglandular connective tissue
3. Largely preventable by prophylactic measures such as good breast hygiene
C. **Assessment findings**
1. Clinical manifestations include:
    a. Elevated temperature, chills
    b. Increased pulse rate
    c. Engorgement, hardness, and reddening of breasts
    d. Nipple soreness, fissures
    e. Swollen, tender axillary lymph nodes
2. Symptoms may occur and the end of the first postpartal week, but most commonly occur in the third or fourth postpartal week.
D. **Nursing diagnoses**
1. Anxiety
2. High Risk for Injury
3. Knowledge Deficit
4. Pain
5. Altered Parenting
5. Anxiety
E. **Planning and implementation**
1. Observe for elevated temperature, chills, tachycardia, headache, pain and tenderness, firmness and redness of breast.
2. Prevent infection through meticulous handwashing technique and prompt attention to blocked milk ducts.
3. Teach mother to breast-feed frequently, adequate breast and nipple care (adequate around-the-clock nonconstrictive support of the breasts, gentleness during care, avoiding harsh cleansing agents and decrusting the nipple, frequent changing

of breast pads, intermittent exposure of nipples to the air), and signs and symptoms of infection.

4. Administer antibiotics and teach mother the importance of following through with prescribed regime even though symptoms have subsided.

5. Provide comfort measures such as small side pillows, icecaps, or heat application over localized abscess.

F. Evaluation

1. The mother verbalizes decrease pain in breasts, can continue nursing infant.

2. The mother demonstrates correct breast hygiene and nursing techniques.

3. The mother verbalizes correct understanding of early signs and symptoms of mastitis.

4. If breast-feeding is discontinued, mother is able to accept the adjustment.

5. The mother follows through with antibiotic regimen.

V. Thrombophlebitis and thrombosis

A. Description

1. Thrombophlebitis in an inflammation of vascular endothelium with clot formation on the vessel wall.

2. Thrombosis formation results when blood components combine to form an aggregate body.

3. Pulmonary embolism occurs when a clot travelling through the venous system becomes lodged within the pulmonary circulatory system, causing occlusion or infarction.

B. Etiology and pathophysiology

1. The incidence of postpartum thrombophlebitis is 0.1% to 1%; when not treated; 24% of these go on to develop pulmonary embolism, with a fatality rate of 15%.

2. Predisposing risk factors include:
   a. History of thrombophlebitis
   b. Obesity
   c. History of cesarean delivery
   d. History of forceps delivery
   e. Older maternal age
   f. Multiparity
   g. Recent infection
   h. Lactation suppression with estrogens
   i. Varicosities
   j. Anemia and blood dyscrasias

C. Assessment findings

1. Superficial thrombophlebitis within the saphenous system presents with midcalf pain, tenderness, redness along the vein.

2. Deep vein thrombosis (DVT) symptoms include muscle pain, swelling, positive Homan's sign, swelling in affected limb.

          3.   Pelvic thrombophlebitis, typically occurring 2 weeks after delivery, is marked by by chills, fever, malaise, and depression.

          4.   Femoral thrombophlebitis, generally occurring 10 days to 2 weeks after delivery, produces chills, fever, malaise, and stiffness and pain of area.

          5.   Pulmonary embolism is heralded by sudden intense chest pain with severe dyspnea followed by tachypnea, pleuritic pain, apprehension, cough, tachycardia, hemoptysis, temperature above 37°C.

D. **Nursing diagnoses**
1. High Risk for Injury
2. Knowledge Deficit
3. Impaired Physical Mobility
4. Pain
5. Altered Parenting
6. Self-care Deficit

E. **Planning and implementation**
1. Monitor vital signs.
2. Assess extremities for signs of inflammation, swelling, positive Homan's sign (pain in the calf on passive dorsiflexion of the foot that may represent a DVT).
3. Teach the patient strategies for preventing venous stasis, such as:
   a. Early ambulation and prevention of pressure on legs
   b. Avoiding standing or sitting for long periods of time
   c. Avoiding crossing legs
4. Administer anticoagulant therapy, as prescribed, and monitor for signs of bleeding and allergic reactions.
5. Keep the antidote protamine sulfate readily available in a dosage of 1 mg/100 U of heparin. (Note: Heparin is incompatible with numerous of antibiotics.)
6. Caution: Do not administer estrogens for lactation suppression, because estrogens may encourage clot formation.
5. Prepare patient for diagnostic studies (i.e., venography and Doppler ultrasound) as indicated.
6. Implement measures to prevent complications of bed rest, as needed (e.g., bed placed in Trendelenburg position, use of footboard, passive or active range of motion, frequent shifts in position, adequate fluid intake and output).
7. Support and communicate with patient and family members during an emergency situation, thus enhancing cooperation with treatment efforts.
8. Provide information regarding treatment regimen (e.g., anticoagulant therapy, analgesics, and bed rest)

F. **Evaluation**
1. The mother is pain free, breathes normally, and returns to stable condition.

2. The mother and family understand events and treatment.
3. The mother is able to continue care of self and infant.

VI. Urinary tract infection (UTI)

A. Description

1. Bacteria defined as the presence of 1,000,000 or more bacterial colonies per milliliter of urine in two consecutive clean, voided, midstream specimens
2. Retention and residual urine: overdistention and incomplete emptying of bladder
3. Cystitis: inflammation of the urinary bladder
4. Pyelonephritis: inflammation of renal pelvis

B. Etiology and pathophysiology

1. UTI occurs in about 5% of postpartum women; increases to 15% of women who have undergone postpartum catheterization.
2. Temporary urine retention may be due to decreased perception of the urge to void due to perineal trauma, and the effects of analgesia or anesthesia.
3. Urinary stasis and residual provides a medium for bacterial growth, predisposing to cystitis and pyelonephritis.
4. Causative organisms in cystitis and pyelonephritis include *Escherichia coli* (most common), *Proteus*, *Pseudomonas*, *Staphylococcus aureus*, and *Streptococcus faecalis*.
5. Consequences of not recognizing early symptoms include the extension of the infection upward with subsequent permanent loss of kidney function.

C. Assessment findings

1. Manifestations of cystitis include frequency, urgency, dysuria, hematuria, nocturia, temperature elevation, and supra pubic pain.
2. Symptoms of pyelonephritis include high temperature, chills, flank pain, nausea, and vomiting.

D. Nursing diagnoses

1. High Risk for Injury
2. Pain
3. Urinary Retention

E. Planning and implementation

1. Obtain specimens, report findings, administer antibiotics and medications.
2. Insert intermittent or indwelling catheter as needed.
3. Note and record response to treatment.
4. Determine if symptoms are present and if woman had difficulty urinating after delivery.
5. Teach self-care related to regular emptying of bladder, proper perineal cleansing, and the need for increased fluids.

F. Evaluation
   1. The mother is able to void and empty bladder.
   2. The mother is able care for self.
   3. The mother is able to follow through with treatment plan.
   4. The mother's urine bacteria colony count decreases to within normal range and symptoms subside.

VII. Postpartum psychosis
   A. Description: three forms of the disorder: postpartum "blues," moderate depression or major affective disorder, and psychotic reaction
   B. Etiology and pathophysiology
      1. Between 50% and 80% of all new mothers report some form of postpartum "blues."
      2. Incidence of moderate depression, or postpartum major affective disorder, ranges from 30 to 200 per 1000 deliveries.
      3. Incidence of puerperal psychosis is approximately one per 1000 live births.
      4. Predisposing factors include previous history of puerperal psychosis, history of manic depressive disorder, delirium and hallucinations, rapid mood change, agitation or confusion; potential for both suicide and infanticide.
   C. Assessment findings
      1. Symptoms associated with postpartum blues include confusion, fatigue, agitation, feelings of hopelessness and shame, and alterations in mood.
      2. Symptoms of postpartum major affective disorder include depression, ambivalence about the pregnancy, feelings of inadequacy, marital discord, guilt and irritability.
      3. Symptoms associated with postpartum psychosis include delusions, auditory hallucinations, and hyperactivity.
   D. Nursing diagnoses
      1. Anxiety
      2. Ineffective Individual and Family Coping
      3. Altered Family Processes
      4. Altered Parenting
   E. Planning and implementation
      1. Provide for continuity of care for mother, newborn, and family.
      2. Develop specific therapeutic goals.
      3. Maintain the prescribed medication schedule.
      4. Provide support for mother's continued care of infant if appropriate and safe for infant.
      5. Keep communication open with health care providers; coordinate social services.
      6. Include family participation and involvement in plans for care.

F. Evaluation
   1. The mother is free of symptoms.
   2. The mother is able to maintain a healthy relationship with the infant and the family.
   3. The mother assumes responsibility for care of infant and herself.

Bibliography

Brunner, L. S., & Suddarth, D. S. (1987). *The Lippincott manual of nursing practice* (4th ed.). Philadelphia: J. B. Lippincott.

Danforth, D. N. (Ed.) (1986). *Obstetrics and gynecology* (5th ed.). Philadelphia: J. B. Lippincott.

Jensen, M. D., & Bobak, I. M. (1985). *Maternity and gynecologic care: The nurse and family* (3rd ed.). St. Louis: C. V. Mosby.

May, K. A., & Mahlmeister, L. R. (1990). *Comprehensive maternity nursing: Nursing process and the childbearing family* (2nd ed.). Philadelphia: J. B. Lippincott.

Olds, S. (1984). *Maternity-newborn nursing.* Menlo Park, CA: Addison-Wesley.

Reeder, S. J., & Martin, L. L. (1987). *Maternity nursing: Family, newborn, and women's health care* (16th ed.). Philadelphia: J. B. Lippincott.

STUDY QUESTIONS

1. Infection of the perineal area (episiotomy site) would exhibit which of the following symptoms?
   a. bruised area and swollen
   b. reddened area and swollen and warm
   c. serous fluid seeping from episiotomy site
   d. bleeding from episiotomy site

2. Mastitis is an infection of the ducts of the breasts. Which of the following organisms is most commonly associated with this infection?
   a. *Staphylococcus aureus*
   b. *Escherichia coli*
   c. *Candida albicans*
   d. HBV virus

3. Which of the following would be the most appropriate nursing action for a postpartal patient diagnosed with thrombophlebitis?
   a. Encourage the patient to walk.
   b. Teach the patient how to massage the painful area.
   c. Encourage bed rest.
   d. Prepare the patient for an extended hospital stay.

4. Mrs. Jones begins hemorrhaging profusely 32 hours after delivery of her second child. The nurse would explain that the probable cause of her hemorrhage is
   a. uterine atony
   b. clotting disorder
   c. laceration
   d. retained placental fragments

5. Mrs. Taylor is 3 days postpartum, following a prolonged labor that ended in a cesarean birth. During assessment, the nurse notes that Mrs. Taylor has an elevated temperature, refused breakfast, and is complaining of a headache, backache, and cramping. Based on these findings, the nurse would be most concerned about which of the following?
   a. retained placental fragments
   b. hemorrhage
   c. mastitis

   d. puerperal infection

6. Prevention of mastitis should be included in the teaching plan for new mothers, if not already done prenatally. Which of the following should *not* be included in the teaching plan?
   a. Observe good handwashing when handling the breasts and nursing.
   b. Wear a tight binder to provide support to the breasts.
   c. Change breast pads frequently.
   d. Expose the breasts to the air periodically.

7. Which of the following data would alert the nurse to the possible presence of deep vein thrombosis in a postpartal patient?
   a. chills, fever, depression, pelvic pressure
   b. chest pain, dyspnea, apprehension
   c. muscle pain, swelling, positive Homan's sign
   d. flank pain, nausea and vomiting, hematuria

8. Which of the following women would be at lowest risk for the development of thrombus or thrombophlebitis?
   a. Susan, age 38 years, who requests lactation suppression in order to return to work
   b. Patty, age 22 years, second birth, vaginal delivery, nursing
   c. Ellen, age 28 years, sixth child, cesarean birth
   d. Martha, age 30 years, third child, 180 lb, forceps delivery

9. Julia Johnson recently gave birth to her first child. She and her husband have looked forward to parenthood eagerly. They attended childbirth education classes and decorated the nursery together, and Julia prepared her body for delivery and nursing with exercise, breathing practice, and breast and nipple toughening. She wanted to be the "perfect mother." But now she has developed a breast abscess and her physi-

cian has advised discontinuation of nursing. Which of the following would most likely be a priority nursing diagnosis for Julia?

a. Altered Patterns of Sexuality related to recent birth

b. Altered Comfort: pain related to breast abscess

c. Disturbance in Self-concept: self-esteem related to disrupted breast-feeding

d. High Risk for Violence: self-directed

10. Mrs. Brown is 2 weeks postpartum. She is ordinarily a healthy functioning wife and mother, but has a history of postpartum depression, having been hospitalized for 2 weeks following the birth of her second child. Now with two children, ages 6 and 4 years, and a new baby, she finds herself tired, angry, and increasingly agitated over day-to-day activities. One day, her husband called the nurse to report that he came home from work just now to find the baby screaming, dirty, and lying on a cluttered tabletop and his wife still in bed. She can't remember where the other two children are and she becomes extremely angry with him, accusing him of "ruining her life." When the nurse arrives at the Brown's home, the husband has found the two older children safe at a neighbor's, the baby is sleeping in his arms, and Mrs. Brown is pacing and shouting how tired she is. Which of the following would likely be the most important immediate intervention?

a. ensuring immediate rest for Mrs. Brown

b. teaching Mrs. Brown about safe, nurturing newborn care

c. protection from harm for Mrs. Brown and for the infant

d. medication for Mrs. Brown to calm her down

ANSWER KEY

202

1. **Correct response: b**
   The infected area usually becomes in-
   flamed, swollen, and warm to touch.
   a. Bruising and swelling do not indi-
      cate infection.
   c. Seeping serous fluid does not indi-
      cate infection.
   d. Bleeding is not normal, but does
      not indicate infection.
   Application/Physiologic/Analysis (Dx)

2. **Correct response: a**
   Staphylococcus aureus is the most common
   causative organism in mastitis.
   b. *Escherichia coli* is a bacteria found in
      lower GI tract.
   c. *Candida albicans* causes monilial in-
      fection.
   d. HBV is associated with hepatitis B.
   Comprehensive/Physiologic/Analysis (Dx)

3. **Correct response: c**
   Activity could dislodge the clot.
   a and b. Ambulation and activity
      could dislodge a clot.
   d. This may occur, but it is not the
      best nursing action.
   Comprehensive/Physiologic/Analysis (Dx)

4. **Correct response: d**
   a and c. Uterine atony and lacerations
      would be causative factors of
      hemorrhage during the first
      24 hours.
   b. A clotting disorder is a possibility,
      but the situation presents no data to
      support this problem.
   Comprehensive/Physiologic/Analysis (Dx)

5. **Correct response: d**
   The data indicate pelvic infection.
   a and b. Retained placenta fragments
      and hemorrhage would re-
      sult in vaginal bleeding.
   c. Mastitis would involve breast in-
      flammation and tenderness.
   Application/Physiologic/Analysis (Dx)

6. **Correct response: b**
   A nonconstrictive bra should be worn
   to support the breasts without binding.

a, c, and d. These are all important
   measures to help prevent
   mastitis.
Comprehensive/Safe care/Planning

7. **Correct response: c**
   Muscle pain, swelling, and positive Homan's sign all point to deep vein thrombosis.
   a. These symptoms are more typical of
      pelvic thrombophlebitis.
   b. These symptoms are more typical of
      pulmonary embolism.
   d. These symptoms are more typical of
      pyelonephritis or urinary tract infec-
      tion.
   Comprehensive/Safe care/Assessment

8. **Correct response: b**
   Patty's young age, second pregnancy,
   vaginal delivery, and nursing place her at
   lowest risk of thrombus or thrombophlebitis.
   a. Susan is at risk because of her age
      and lactation suppression.
   c. Ellen is at risk because of multiparity
      and history of cesarean delivery.
   d. Martha is at risk because of obesity
      and forceps delivery.
   Application/Safe care/Assessment

9. **Correct response: c**
   Based on Julia's high hopes for and
   preparation for breast-feeding, this diagnosis likely would be the highest priority.
   a and b. Although these could be cur-
      rent diagnoses on this pa-
      tient's care plan, they are not
      as high a priority to Julia as
      her feelings about not being
      able to breast-feed her infant
      as she planned.
   d. There are no data to support sui-
      cidal potential.
   Application/Psychosocial/Analysis (Dx)

10. **Correct response: c**
    The baby and Mrs. Brown are at risk be-
    cause of her depressed and psychotic be-

havior, warranting pharmacologic intervention.

a and d. Mrs. Brown requires more
assistance than rest and medication.

b. She is too out of control for teaching to be helpful.

Application/Safe care/Planning

Neonatal Complications

I. Overview

A. Essential concepts

1. Early identification of the high-risk newborns is the first step in monitoring for and intervening in complications to reduce morbidity and mortality.

    2. Major complications of newborns covered in this chapter include:

        a. Birth asphyxia

        b. Complications related to gestational age: preterm, small-for-gestational age (SGA), large-for-gestational age (LGA), post-term.

    3. Other complications not covered in this chapter include:

        a. Birth injuries (e.g., fractures of skull, clavicle, humerus, or femur)

        b. Infection: bacterial, viral, protozoal

        c. Hemolytic disease: Rh and ABO incompatibility

        d. Central nervous system injuries (e.g., intracranial hemorrhage, brachial plexus injury, facial nerve injury, phrenic nerve injury)

        e. Maternal substance abuse (e.g., alcohol, cocaine)

B. **General nursing management of the high-risk newborn**

    1. Assessment

        a. Sources of data: maternal and neonatal health histories, systematic physical and behavioral assessments

        b. Initial assessment to screen for risk factors

        c. Ongoing assessment of the high-risk newborn

    2. Nursing diagnoses: in addition to complication-specific nursing diagnoses, the following diagnoses are common to care of high-risk newborns:

        a. High Risk for Altered Body Temperature

        b. Fluid Volume Deficit

        c. Impaired Gas Exchange

        d. High Risk for Infection

        e. Altered Nutrition: Less than Body Requirements

        f. Altered Parenting

    3. Planning and implementation

        a. Support cardiopulmonary adaptation; maintain adequate airway.

        b. Administer oxygen using oxygen mask, endotracheal tube, oxygen hood or nasal prongs.

        c. Support ventilatory capacity.

        d. Promote fluid and electrolyte balance.

        e. Provide for nutritional needs.

        f. Prevent infection.

        g. Support thermoregulation.

        h. Promote behavioral adaptation and parent–newborn attachment.

        i. Monitor for potential complications related to oxygen toxicity (e.g., retinopathy prematurity and bronchopulmonary dysplasia).

        j.   Monitor for the potential complications of hyperbilirubin-emia and kernicterus.

        k.   Support conjugation and excretion of bilirubin.

        l.   Monitor for possibility of altered parenting.

   4. Evaluation

        a.   The neonate achieves and maintains normal cardiac output and adequate tissue perfusion.

        b.   Normal respiratory pattern and adequate gas exchange is achieved and maintained.

        c.   Fluid and electrolyte balance is achieved.

        d.   Nutritional requirements for growth and development are maintained.

        e.   The newborn remains free of infection.

        f.   Newborn maintains normal core temperature.

        g.   Newborn achieves a state of behavioral stabilization and beginning organization.

        h.   Newborn undergoing oxygen therapy demonstrates absence of oxygen toxicity as evidenced by normal arterial blood gas (ABG) values.

        i.   Newborn undergoing phototherapy responds with reduced hyperbilirubinemia.

        j.   Newborn receiving exchange transfusion remains free of complications and maintains serum bilirubin levels within normal limits.

II. Birth asphyxia

  A. **Description: a condition characterized by hypoxemia (decreased PaO_2), hypercarbia (increased $PaCO_2$), and acidosis (lowered pH).**

  B. **Etiology and incidence**

    1. Causative factors can include:

       a.   Impaired maternal blood flow through the placenta

       b.   Impaired blood flow through the umbilical cord

       c.   Impaired fetal circulation

       d.   Impaired respiratory effort

    2. Unless vigorous resuscitation is started promptly, irreversible changes in brain and myocardial tissues will occur, possibly leading to permanent brain damage or death.

    3. During the 24 hours following successful resuscitation, the neonate is vulnerable for the development of postasphyxial syndrome.

  C. **Assessment**

    1. Clinical signs of birth asphyxia include:

       a.   Increased PaO_2 level

       b.   Increased $PaCO_2$

       c.   Low pH

       d.   Minimal or absent respiratory effort

        e.   Depressed cardiac function

      2.   The newborn may gasp for breath in an attempt to inflate the lungs.

  D. **Nursing diagnoses**

      1.   Ineffective Breathing Pattern

      2.   Impaired Gas Exchange

  E. **Planning and implementation**

      1.   Observe newborn who has been successfully resuscitated for the following constellation of signs:

          a.   Seizure activity within the first 24 hours after birth

          b.   Necrosis of both renal and intestinal tissues

          c.   Metabolic alterations (e.g., hypoglycemia, hypocalcemia, hyperkalemia)

          d.   Increased intracranial pressure, marked by bulging fontanels, "setting sun" eyes, decreased or absent reflexes, and seizures

          e.   Myocardial ischemia (dysrhythmias), intestinal ischemia, and necrotizing enterocolitis (absence of bowel sounds, increasing girth, and bloody stools)

      2.   Maintain the neonate's gut in a resting state by keeping the neonate NPO for at least 24 to 48 hours.

      3.   Record and monitor intake and output to evaluate renal function and rule out renal failure.

      4.   Check every voiding for presence of blood and protein, suggesting renal injury.

      5.   Check every stool for blood, suggesting necrotizing enterocolitis.

      6.   Facilitate serial blood glucose determinations to detect hypoglycemia and serum electrolytes, once or twice daily, to detect hypocalcemia and hyperkalemia, as ordered.

      7.   Maintain intravenous fluids.

      8.   Administer antibiotics and seizure medications (e.g., Dilantin, phenobarbital), as ordered.

      9.   Support parents in dealing with the uncertainties of long-term neurologic functioning.

  F. **Evaluation**

      1.   Complications of postasphyxial syndrome are identified early and appropriate interventions maintained.

      2.   Neonate responds to treatment for seizure activity, as evidenced by normalization of neurologic and physiologic status and absence of recurrent seizure activity.

      3.   Parents verbalize accurate understanding of the neonate's condition and prognosis.

III. **Preterm newborn**

  A. **Description: neonate born before 37 weeks' gestation**

  B. **Etiology and pathophysiology**

      1.   The etiology of preterm labor is poorly understood.

2. Among the many possible contributing factors are:
   a. Premature rupture of the membranes
   b. Preeclampsia
   c. Hydramnios
   d. Placenta previa
   e. Abruptio placentae
   f. Incompetent cervix
   g. Trauma
   h. Uterine structural anomalies
   i. Congenital adrenal hyperplasia
   j. Fetal death
3. Maternal risk factors include age under 18 years, history of preterm labors, multiple pregnancy, hydramnios, smoking, poor hygiene, poor nutrition, employment.
4. Preterm newborns exhibit anatomic and physiologic immaturity in all body systems; this immaturity hinders many of the major adaptations to extrauterine life that the newborn must make.

C. Assessment findings
   1. Respiratory status: tachypnea, grunting, nasal flaring, retraction, cyanosis
   2. Cardiovascular status: decreased oxygen saturation, decreased oxygen levels, abnormal ABGs
   3. Gastrointestinal status: decreased gag, suck, and swallow; gastric reflux; vomiting; gastric residuals; weight loss; failure to gain 10 to 15 g/day
   4. Fluid status
      a. Excess: edema, congestive heart failure
      b. Deficit: tachycardia, poor skin turgor, decreased urine output, abnormal electrolyte levels, increased urine osmolarity (pH), decreased blood pressure
   5. Physiologic anemia: tachycardia, pallor, decreased blood pressure, apnea, failure to gain weight
   6. Signs and symptoms of neonatal infection: temperature instability; hypothermia; apnea; cyanosis; decreased oxygen saturation; poor feeding; gastric residuals
   7. Hypoglycemia or hyperglycemia
   8. Temperature control: unstable body core temperature
   9. Neuromuscular system status: arching behaviors, hyperextension of extremities, resistance to cuddling
   10. Altered parenting:
       a. Decreased or absent parental visits
       b. Resistance or refusal of parents to participate in newborn care
       c. Denial of severity of newborn illness
       d. Resistance or refusal to touch newborn
       e. Persistent verbalization of guilt

D. **Nursing diagnoses**
1. Ineffective Airway Clearance
2. Ineffective Breathing Patterns
3. Fluid Volume Excess/Fluid Volume Deficit
4. Impaired Gas Exchange
5. Hypothermia
6. High Risk for Infection
7. Impaired Physical Mobility
8. Altered Nutrition: Less than Body Requirements
9. Altered Parenting

E. **Planning and implementation**
1. Maintain a patent airway
   a. Suction the newborn as indicated
   b. Position the newborn on abdomen or side, or with a small pillow under the head and shoulders to maintain airway.
   c. Position the newborn to facilitate drainage of mucus or regurgitated milk.
2. Support respiratory efforts:
   a. Electronically monitor breathing and heart rate.
   b. Prevent gastric distention by aspirating air before gavage feedings and avoiding overfeeding.
   c. Discontinue oral feeding if respiratory distress occurs.
   d. Administer oxygen concentrations to keep PO_2 between 50 to 80 mmHg on ABGs
3. Monitor ambient oxygen concentration with an oxygen analyzer; use a $TcPO_2$ monitor or an oxygen saturation monitor (pulse oximetry).
4. Provide appropriate nutrition.
   a. Administer correct formula in correct amounts.
   b. Check for residual before gavage feeding.
   c. Measure abdominal girth every 4 hours.
5. Evaluate for evidence of exhaustion during feeding.
   a. Maintain neutral thermal environment and normal body temperature.
   b. Obtain weight daily, and plot on growth chart.
   c. Test all stools for glucose.
6. Prevent and monitor for development of necrotizing enterocolitis (NEC) by:
   a. Testing all stools for presence of occult blood
   b. Positioning the newborn on the right side after feeding to promote stomach emptying
   c. Avoiding disturbing the newborn for at least 1 hour after feeding to facilitate stomach emptying and nutrient absorption
7. Prevent and monitor for fluid volume excess by:
   a. Meticulously monitoring intake and output

b. Administering diuretics as ordered

c. Regulating all intravenous infusions with an intravenous infusion pump

d. Administering proper solutions and formulas

8. Prevent and monitor for fluid volume deficit by:

a. Assessing daily sodium, chloride, and potassium levels

b. Minimizing insensible water losses: cover the newborn with a heat shield, humidify oxygen, close isolette ports

c. Minimizing withdrawal of blood for laboratory analysis

d. Testing all voidings for pH and specific gravity

9. Prevent and monitor for physiologic anemia by:

a. Minimizing withdrawal of blood for laboratory analysis

b. Administering vitamin K to prevent hemorrhagic disease of the newborn

c. Placing the newborn in a neutral thermal environment to decrease energy requirements in case of severe anemia

10. Prevent and monitor for metabolic alterations by checking blood sugar levels using Dextrostix or Chemstrip for evidence of hypoglycemia or hyperglycemia.

11. Prevent hypothermia and cold stress by placing the newborn in a neutral thermal environment.

12. Observe for skin jaundice and signs and symptoms of bilirubin encephalopathy.

13. Place the newborn prone with flexed extremities close to the body; encourage flexion in the supine position by using blanket rolls.

14. Provide the newborn with body boundaries through swaddling or using blanket rolls against the newborn's body and feet.

15. Develop an appropriate newborn stimulation plan based on gestational age, physiologic limitations, and presence of disease.

16. Monitor for altered parenting and facilitate parental attachment by:

a. Encouraging early and frequent visits by parents

b. Placing name on newborn's isolette

c. Providing parents with the unit phone number and names of staff caring for the neonate

d. Giving parents the opportunity to provide progressively complex care for the newborn

e. Pointing out the newborn's unique characteristics

F. **Evaluation**

1. The preterm neonate establishes respiratory function, as evidenced by successful weaning from mechanical support by the time of discharge.

2. The preterm neonate gains weight and shows no signs of gastrointestinal complications.

3. The preterm newborn achieves fluid and electrolyte balance, as

evidenced by output of 1 to 3 mL/kg/hour in the first week of life.

4. The preterm newborn maintains hematocrit level of 10 g/dL.
5. The preterm newborn remains free of metabolic alterations.
6. The preterm newborn maintains a normal core temperature, as evidenced by axillary temperature of 36.4°C to 37.2°C.
7. The preterm newborn remains free of hyperbilirubinemia or encephalopathy.
8. The preterm newborn develops increasingly organized patterns of behavior and demonstrates age-appropriate growth and development.
9. Parents of the preterm newborn demonstrate appropriate and progressive attachment behaviors (e.g., frequent visits or calls, increasing interest and confidence in providing care, calling the newborn by name).

IV. SGA newborn

A. Description: a newborn whose weight falls below the tenth percentile or is two standard deviations below the mean as a result of intrauterine growth retardation (IUGR)

B. Etiology and pathophysiology

1. Predisposing factors: maternal malnutrition, premature placental aging secondary to diabetes mellitus or other vascular conditions, placental infarcts, congenital infections, teratogens, and maternal substance abuse
2. In symmetrical IUGR, the fetus experiences early and prolonged nutritional deprivation caused by severe chronic maternal malnutrition, placental insufficiency, intrauterine infection, or fetal chromosomal anomalies; characterized by:
   a. Hypoplastic cell growth and development
   b. Head circumference below tenth percentile
   c. Diminished brain size and permanent mental retardation
3. Asymmetrical IUGR results from nutritional deficits and placental insufficiency in late pregnancy; characterized by:
   a. Diminished cell size but not cell numbers
   b. Disproportionately large head in relation to body, with long and emaciated trunk and little subcutaneous fat
   c. Head circumference approaching norm
4. In asymmetrical IUGR, postnatal growth and development are rapid and the potential for normal intellectual functioning is excellent.

C. Assessment findings

1. Respiratory status and breathing pattern: tachypnea, grunting, flaring, retractions, cyanosis, decreased oxygen saturation, abnormal ABGs
2. Physical features and growth status: dysmorphic features; wasting of trunk and extremities; rough, dry skin; large anterior fontanel

      3. Nutritional status: gastric reflux, weight loss, failure to gain weight (10 to 15 g/day)

      4. Metabolic status: jitteriness, lethargy, cyanosis, apnea, Dextrostix or Chemstrip equal to or less than 45 mg/dL

      5. Hematologic status: hematocrit >65%, plethora, cyanosis, respiratory distress, central nervous system (CNS) aberrations (lethargy, poor feeding, convulsions, hypotonia), hypoglycemia

      6. Unstable temperature control: temperature swings; temperature equal to or less than 36.4°C

D. **Nursing diagnoses**

      1. Ineffective Airway Clearance

      2. Ineffective Breathing Pattern

      3. Ineffective Gas Exchange

      4. Altered Growth and Development

      5. Hypothermia

      6. Altered Nutrition: Less than Body requirements

E. **Planning and implementation**

      1. Support airway clearance by suctioning as needed, administering humidified mist to liquefy secretions, perform chest physiotherapy to facilitate drainage.

      2. Monitor and support breathing patterns by electronically monitoring cardiopulmonary status, positioning to facilitate chest expansion, preventing stomach distention (e.g., avoid overfeeding and aspirating air before gavage feeding).

      3. Promote effective gas exchange by administering oxygen concentrations to maintain PO_2 at 60 to 80 mmHg and monitoring concentrations with a $PtCO_2$ monitor or O_2 monitor.

      4. Assess prenatal history for possible TORCH (toxoplasmosis, rubella, cytomegalovirus, and herpes simplex) infections during pregnancy or maternal substance abuse; assess IgM levels which, if elevated, could point to intrauterine infection.

      5. Provide small frequent feedings to accommodate the SGA newborn's small stomach capacity; obtain daily weights and plot them on a growth chart.

      6. Assess for evidence of hypoglycemia at birth, hourly until stable, and before feedings.

      7. Obtain central hematocrit at birth to evaluate for hyperviscosity; be alert for ischemia of organs, thrombus formation, hypoglycemia and respiratory distress associated with polycythemia.

      8. Maintain a neutral thermal environment.

F. **Evaluation**

      1. The SGA newborn maintains optimal respiratory and cardiac function.

      2. The SGA newborn demonstrates age-appropriate growth and development by discharge.

3. The SGA newborn begins to gain weight and length and to approximate normal newborn parameters.
4. The SGA newborn maintains a normal core temperature, as evidenced by an axillary temperature of 36.4°C to 37.2°C.

V. LGA newborn

A. **Description: a newborn with birth weight over 4000 g or above the 90th percentile or two standard deviations above the mean**

B. **Etiology and pathophysiology**
1. Predisposing factors: genetic predisposition, excessive maternal weight gain during pregnancy, maternal gestational diabetes
2. An infant of a diabetic mother (IDM) commonly is LGA due to high levels of maternal glucose that cross the placenta during pregnancy (IDM with vascular changes may also be SGA due to decreased placental functioning).
3. LGA newborns are at risk for:
    a. Hypoglycemia due to limited liver glycogen stores
    b. Polycythemia due to chronic intrauterine hypoxia, which causes increased red blood cell (RBC) production
    c. Birth injuries due to disproportionate size of newborn to birth passageway

C. **Assessment findings**
1. Prenatal history may reveal maternal diabetes mellitus.
2. The newborn may exhibit signs and symptoms of hypoglycemia: Dextrostix or Chemstrip value equal to or less than 45 mg/dL, tremors, hypotonia, lethargy, irritability, apnea, seizures (relevant for SGA IDM as well).
3. The LGA newborn is prone to complications of birth injury, such as:
    a. Fractured clavicle: crepitus, hematoma, or deformity over clavicle, decreased movement of arm on the affected side, asymmetrical or absent Moro reflex
    b. Bell's palsy: facial hemiparesis, evidenced by drooping of lip to normal side, no wrinkling of forehead on affected side
    c. Erb-Duchenne palsy, or brachial plexus paralysis: one arm weakness or paralysis; weak or absent grip
    d. Phrenic nerve palsy: weakness of the diaphragm with possible dyspnea, decreased breath sounds in lower lobes, and poor to absent rise of the abdomen with inspiration
    e. Possible skull fracture: soft tissue swelling over site of fracture; visible indentation in scalp; cephalhematoma; positive skull radiograph; CNS signs with intracranial hemorrhage (e.g., lethargy, seizures, apnea, hypotonia)
3. Hyperthermia may develop due to increased amount of fatty tissue serving as insulation

D. **Nursing diagnoses**
  1. Altered Growth and Development
  2. Hyperthermia
  3. High Risk for Injury
E. **Planning and implementation**
  1. Monitor for and prevent hypoglycemia by:
      a. Check Dextrostix or Chemstrip every 30 minutes four times; every hour until feedings are started; then, before each feeding until the newborn is stable.
      b. Administer D5W by mouth using nipple or gavage.
      c. Retest blood glucose less than 15 minutes after feeding.
      d. Notify the physician of decreased blood glucose readings.
      e. Begin oral formula or breast-feeding as soon as possible.
  2. If IDM, observe for potential complications (SGA, LGA) and possible complications (e.g., hypocalcemia, respiratory distress syndrome [RDS], polycythemia, undiagnosed congenital anomalies or heart murmur, altered parenting).
  3. Observe for complications of birth injury.
F. **Evaluation**
  1. The LGA newborn responds to appropriate support and demonstrates no signs of hypoglycemia.
  2. The LGA newborn makes the transition to extrauterine life without sequelae or with resolution of sequelae within a few days or weeks after birth.
  3. The LGA newborn maintains normal temperature, as evidenced by axillary temperature of 36.4°C to 37.2°C.
  4. Parents of the LGA newborn demonstrate signs of growing attachment to the newborn as evidenced by their participation in care and growing ease in handling the newborn.

VI. **Post-term newborn**
  A. **Description: a neonate born after 42 weeks' gestation**
  B. **Etiology and pathophysiology**
  1. Factors associated with postmaturity include first pregnancies, grand multiparity, history of prolonged pregnancy, anencephaly, trisomy 16 to 18, Seckel's dwarfism.
  2. Mortality rate is twice that of full-term newborns.
  3. The newborn is at increased risk for developing complications related to compromised uteroplacental perfusion and hypoxia (e.g., meconium aspiration syndrome [MAS], pneumothorax, and potential complications of hypoglycemia, polycythemia, and hypothermia)
  C. **Assessment findings**
  1. Characteristics: long thin newborn with wasted appearance, parchment-like skin, meconium-stained skin, nails, and umbilical cord as a result of intrauterine hypoxia

      2. MAS is manifested by fetal hypoxia, meconium staining of amniotic fluid, respiratory distress at delivery, meconium-stained vocal cords.

      3. The newborn may exhibit signs of pneumothorax: acute respiratory distress (tachypnea, flaring, grunting, retraction) cyanosis or pallor, skin mottling, decreased PaO_2, asymmetrical chest expansion, possible diminished breath sounds on affected side, cardiovascular changes

D. **Nursing diagnoses**
      1. Ineffective Breathing Pattern
      2. Impaired Gas Exchange
      3. Altered Growth and Development
      4. Hypothermia

E. **Planning and implementation**
      1. When assisting with birth of a post-term newborn with meconium-stained amniotic fluid, be prepared to suction the trachea, visualize the cords, and support respiratory efforts.
          a. Respiratory assistance using mechanical ventilation
          b. Maintenance of a neutral thermal environment
          c. Chest physiotherapy, postural drainage
          d. Administration of antibiotics
          e. Administration of a vasodilator if indicated to correct pulmonary hypertension
          f. Maintenance of extracorporeal membrane oxygenation if indicated to correct persistent pulmonary hypertension
      2. Ongoing care of an uncomplicated post-term neonate focuses on observation and support of respiratory function and prevention of complications; includes:
          a. Serial glucose monitoring
          b. Early feeding to prevent hypogylcemia if not contraindicated by respiratory status
      3. If pneumothorax occurs, emergency aspiration and chest tube insertion may be indicated, followed by continuous monitoring of respiratory status.

F. **Evaluation**
      1. The post-term newborn progresses and stabilizes with no untoward sequelae.
      2. Complications of postmaturity are identified early, with prompt interventions that support the newborn's transition to extrauterine life, with resolution of sequelae within a few days or weeks of birth.
      3. Parents of the post-term newborn demonstrate understanding of their newborn's condition and care.

Bibliography

Brunner, L. S., & Suddarth, D. S. (1987). *The Lippincott manual of nursing practice* (4th ed.). Philadelphia: J. B. Lippincott.

Danforth, D. N. (Ed.) (1986). *Obstetrics and gynecology* (5th ed.). Philadelphia: J. B. Lippincott.

Jensen, M. D., & Bobak, I. M. (1985). *Maternity and gynecologic care: The nurse and family* (3rd ed.). St. Louis: C. V. Mosby.

May, K. A., & Mahlmeister, L. R. (1990). *Comprehensive maternity nursing: Nursing process and the childbearing family* (2nd ed.). Philadelphia: J. B. Lippincott.

Olds, S. (1984). *Maternity-newborn nursing*. Menlo Park, CA: Addison-Wesley.

Reeder, S. J., & Martin, L. L. (1987). *Maternity nursing: Family, newborn, and women's health care* (16th ed.). Philadelphia: J. B. Lippincott.

STUDY QUESTIONS

1. While in labor, Beverly Thomas, a 37-year-old primipara, tells the nurse she had a brother with Down's syndrome who died when he was 2 years old because of a heart defect. She states she is concerned that this pregnancy could also result in the birth of an affected child who will die. She has had no genetic counseling. It would be most appropriate if the nurse initiated which of the following at this time?
   a. Refer her and her partner to the geneticist on call.
   b. Notify the nursery of an impending affected baby.
   c. Explore and document parental wishes for the level of aggressiveness of management they would desire.
   d. Allow her to express her concerns without discounting her fears.

2. Lisa, 32 years old and in the 26th week of pregnancy, has been told by her primary care provider that sonogram shows an abnormal amount of fluid surrounding her fetus. With further exploration, the nurse determines that Lisa has hydramnios, a condition often associated with which of the following?
   a. urinary tract anomalies such as renal agenesis and renal stenosis
   b. hydrocephalus, cleft lip, Down's syndrome, and pyloric stenosis
   c. trisomy 21, 31 and Klinefelter's syndrome
   d. inborn errors of metabolism

3. Mrs. Kline delivered a 42-week gestation, 6.4-lb male newborn 45 minutes ago. Following a period of increasing respiratory distress, the pediatrician suspects a diaphragmatic hernia. The nurse is aware that this is a surgical emergency and that the baby will be immediately transported by to a regional center for corrective surgery. In preparing the family for separation, it is most important that the nurse
   a. Shelter the parents from contact with the newborn so they will not become attached.
   b. Ensure privacy and plenty of opportunity for family members to express their sadness and guilt.
   c. Reassure them that everything will be all right because the team is well prepared and the newborn's Apgar score was 5 and 10 at birth.
   d. Keep them informed about what is transpiring relative to their newborn and provide as much opportunity for parent–newborn contact as the newborn's condition allows.

4. In planning care for a cyanotic newborn suspected of having a diaphragmatic hernia during the hour immediately following birth, the nurse's priority would be focused on which of the following?
   a. assisting in the establishment of an umbilical catheter line
   b. attaching the newborn bracelet and obtaining footprints in preparation for transport to surgery
   c. assisting to establish adequate ventilation and oxygenation
   d. placing the newborn on the affected side to allow for normal lung expansion

5. When caring for a 23-year-old, cocaine-addicted mother in labor at an estimated 30th week of gestation, the nurse's primary initial concern relative to providing appropriate care to the fetus is which of the following?
   a. the imminent birth of a preterm newborn with RDS
   b. the possibility of cerebral infarction or placental abruption in addition to a preterm birth
   c. observation for the predictable sequence of heroin-like symptoms of withdrawal
   d. The most worrisome symptoms in cocaine-addicted neonates do not appear until they are school aged.

6. When reviewing the prenatal history of

Vivian Shore, a 19-year-old gravida 5, para 3, the nurse notes that Vivian's prenatal care consisted of two antepartum visits, one at 14 weeks and the second at 25 weeks, where she tested positive for HIV. She is in active labor at 40 weeks' gestation. The nurse would expect the newborn to be infected with the virus based on observation of which of the following?
a. strawberry-red color to skin; patches of pustules over the trunk
b. simian creases in both hands, polydactyly, imperforate anus
c. SGA, birth weight 2200 g; eyes mildly oblique, patulous lips
d. respiratory distress within 30 minutes; Grade IV diastolic murmur

7. The nurse palpates for the liver and spleen of an HIV-infected neonate and determines that the liver is palpable at 1 cm below the right costal margin but that the spleen is not palpable. The newborn is lethargic, and capillary refill time is 5 seconds. These findings are consistent with which of the following nursing diagnoses?
a. Impaired Gas Exchange related to invasion of the immune system through infecting helper T cells
b. Altered Nutrition: Less Than Body Requirements related to poor feeding
c. High Risk for Infection related to abnormal immunoregulation
d. Sensory Alteration related to CNS changes

8. In assessing the newborn with jaundiced skin tone 6 hours after birth, the nurse would review the perinatal record for any conditions associated with RBC destruction. Such conditions could include all of the following *except*

a. perinatal asphyxia with a pH less than 7.2, Apgar of 3 or less at 5 minutes; hypothermia ($>35°C$ or 95°F)
b. phenylketonuria
c. Rh − mother; positive Coombs test
d. yellow-stained vernix or umbilical cord

9. G6PD is characterized by a deficiency of a sex-linked red blood cell enzyme (G6PD); this abnormality is found in 10% of the black population. The affected chromosome is carried on the X (female) chromosome. In caring for a woman in labor whose prenatal history reveals G6PD deficiency, the nurse would be concerned that the newborn would be at risk for which of the following?
a. respiratory distress syndrome, death
b. neonatal jaundice, erythroblastosis fetalis, death
c. hemolytic disease of the newborn, splenomegaly
d. urinary tract infection or anomalies

10. Approximately 250,000 newborns are born each year with significant structural and functional disorders; 1% of all newborns have congenital anomalies severe enough to require surgery to avoid death. The most common surgical emergencies during the newborn period are which of the following?
a. meningomyelocele, megacolon, coanal atresia
b. congenital heart defects such as VSD, ASD, and hyperplastic left heart
c. diaphragmatic hernia, tracheoesophageal atresia, omphalocele, intestinal obstruction, imperforate anus
d. pyloric stenosis, cleft palate, volvulus, deformed extremities

ANSWER KEY

1. *Correct response: d*
Based on the situation, providing emotional support would be most appropriate.
  a. This would be most appropriate during the prenatal period.
  b. The newborn may be affected, but the risk is not sufficient to put everyone on extra alert.
  c. This would be appropriate if there were other data suggesting a poor outcome (e.g., hydramnios).
Analysis/Health promotion/Implementation

2. *Correct response: b*
Hydramnios is associated with hydrocephalus, cleft lip, Down's syndrome, and pyloric stenosis.
  a. This is associated with oligohydramnios, decreased amounts of amniotic fluid.
  c and d. These conditions are not associated with abnormal amounts of amniotic fluid.
Comprehensive/Psychological/Analysis (Dx)

3. *Correct response: d*
Keeping the parents informed and encouraging parent–infant bonding can help ease the stress associated with separation.
  a. Parents of compromised newborns need an opportunity to touch and smell and see their newborn, especially when they will be separated.
  b. This would be most appropriate during a later period in the grieving process.
  c. This is inappropriate because the nurse does not know whether the newborn will be all right, and the Apgar is not a relevant measure of how an newborn with diaphragmatic hernia will progress.
Application/Psychosocial/Implementation

4. *Correct response: c*
Establishing adequate ventilation and oxygenation is the initial priority for this infant.

  a and b. These may be indicated but are not priority issues.
  d. This is indicated in the presence of atelectasis.
Analysis/Safe care/Planning

5. *Correct response: b*
This patient is at risk for preterm birth, cerebral infarction, and placental abruption.
  a. Although concerned about a preterm birth, the nurse must observe for signs of abruption and CNS symptoms associated with perinatal cerebral infarction.
  c. Cocaine-addicted newborns do not exhibit the predictable sequence of physical withdrawal associated with heroin.
  d. Although it is true that some newborns remain asymptomatic at birth and do not exhibit symptoms of fetal cocaine addiction until later, this would not be the most urgent concern during the perinatal period.
Analysis/Safe care/Analysis (Dx)

6. *Correct response: c*
SGA, oblique eyes, and patulous lips may point to HIV infection in a high-risk infant.
  a, b, and d. These are not associated specifically with newborns infected in utero with the AIDS virus, although a newborn with AIDS may have these symptoms as well.
Analysis/Physiologic/Analysis (Dx)

7. *Correct response: c*
The signs and symptoms point to the nursing diagnosis High Risk for Infection.
  a, b, and d. These could also be relevant nursing diagnoses for the HIV infected neonate; however, the signs and symptoms presented in the question

are relevant to the new-
born's increased susceptibility for infection.
Application/Safe care/Analysis (Dx)

8. *Correct response: b*
   G6PD, not phenylketonuria, is associated with overproduction of unconjugated bilirubin.
   a, c, and d. These are all signs or
   symptoms of the possi-
   bility of increased RBC
   destruction.
Analysis/Physiologic/Assessment

9. *Correct response: b*
   The newborn of a mother with G6PD
   deficiency is at increased risk for neona-

tal jaundice, erythroblastosis fetalis, and
death.
   a and c. These responses are only partially correct.
   d. This is a maternal risk only.
Analysis/Safe care/Analysis (Dx)

10. *Correct response: c*
    This list includes the most common sur-
    gical emergencies in the newborn.
    a, b, and d. These are lists of rela-
    tively common disorders,
    but at least one disorder
    in each list would not be
    considered an emer-
    gency, life-threatening
    problem.
Comprehensive/Physiologic/Planning

1. Sue, a 25-year-old primigravida at 20 weeks' gestation, during a routine prenatal visit complained of swelling and pain in her "private area." Upon examination, you find that there is a red swollen area 23 cm in size on the right side of her vaginal orifice. Upon examination it was found that Sue had an enlarged
   a. Bartholin's gland
   b. clitoris
   c. parotid gland
   d. Skene's gland

2. The raised longitudinal folds of pigmented adipose tissue containing hair that extends from the mons veneris to the perineum is called the
   a. labia minora
   b. labia majora
   c. mons pubis
   d. vestibule

3. It was determined that Sue had a platypelloid pelvis. You know that this pelvis is
   a. a typical female pelvis with rounded inlet
   b. a normal male pelvis with heart-shaped inlet
   c. an ape-like pelvis with an oval inlet
   d. a flat female pelvis with a transverse oval inlet

4. When examining Sue's abdomen, you find that the tip of the uterus is 20 cm above the symphysis pubis. The upper rounded portion of the uterus is the
   a. corpus
   b. decidua
   c. fundus
   d. isthmus

5. When measuring the pelvic inlet, it was found that the obstetric conjugate was 10 cm. This indicates that the anteroposterior diameter is
   a. within normal limits for a normal vaginal delivery

b. too narrow for normal vaginal delivery
   c. considered to be extremely large
   d. considered to be marginal

6. If the embryo is to differentiate as a female, what hormonal stimulation must occur?
   a. an increase in maternal estrogen secretion
   b. a decrease in maternal androgen secretion
   c. secretion of androgen by the fetal gonad
   d. secretion of estrogen by the fetal gonad

7. Ann is pregnant for the third time. She has a little girl 3 years of age and had a spontaneous abortion at 16 weeks' gestation. Which of the following is correct regarding the gravida and para of Ann?
   a. gravida 2, para 1
   b. gravida 2, para 2
   c. gravida 3, para 1
   d. gravida 3, para 2

8. Ann had a pregnancy test to determine if she was pregnant. The hormone responsible for the positive pregnancy test is
   a. human chorionic gonadotropin
   b. estrogen
   c. follicle-stimulating hormone
   d. progesterone

9. Ann has experienced amenorrhea, nausea, urinary frequency, and breast tenderness. These changes are known as
   a. expected changes
   b. presumptive changes
   c. probable changes
   d. positive changes

10. Upon pelvic examination, it was noted that Ann's cervix was a blue-purple color. This is called
    a. Braxton's sign
    b. Chadwick's sign
    c. Goodell's sign
    d. McDonald's sign

Answer sheet provided on page 235.

11. A client in the antepartal clinic complains of feeling faint while lying in a dorsal recumbent position. Your reaction would be to
   a. Help the woman up into a sitting position.
   b. Help the woman to turn on her left side in Sim's position.
   c. Get the woman a drink of water.
   d. Notify the doctor immediately.

12. During the prenatal visit, a woman complained of a sudden grabbing pain in the calf of her leg while lying on the examination table. Which of the following actions should the nurse take?
   a. Massage her calf.
   b. Place a warm compress on her calf.
   c. Dorsiflex her foot and press her knee downward.
   d. Elevate her leg until the pain subsides.

13. The patient states that the doctor said there was "ballottement present." She asks, "What does this mean?" The nurse should explain that ballottement is the
   a. examiner's palpation of contractions
   b. fetal movements felt by the mother
   c. passive movement of the unengaged fetus
   d. enlargement and softening of the uterus

14. The nurse examines the woman's breasts during a prenatal clinic visit. Which of the following findings must be reported to the physician?
   a. tenderness
   b. prominent superficial veins
   c. increased pigmentation of areola and nipple
   d. nodularity in the upper left outer quadrant

15. Mary asked the nurse when she should gain the most weight in pregnancy. Which of the following responses by the nurse would be best?
   a. "Normally, weight is gained equally in each of the three trimesters."
   b. "Most weight is gained equally in the last two trimesters."

   c. "Most women gain too much in the first trimester and then try to decrease their gain in the second and third trimesters."
   d. "Most weight is gained (about 1 lb/week) during the last two trimesters."

16. Mary asked the nurse, "The doctor wanted me to have a sonogram test next week. Why is this extra expense necessary?" The nurse's best response would be which of the following?
   a. "We want to determine the sex of the child so you can plan for him or her."
   b. "It is important to determine the approximate date (within 2 weeks) of expected delivery."
   c. "This is a common practice due to the increasing number of lawsuits brought against obstetricians."
   d. "This is a way to diagnose early fetal anomalies."

17. Mary told the nurse that the only discomfort she had noticed was slight nausea for part of the morning. Which of the following would be an *inappropriate* response by the nurse?
   a. "Bicarbonate of soda, 1 teaspoon in 8 oz of water, will decrease nausea."
   b. "Eating a few low-sodium crackers will often decrease the nausea."
   c. "Avoid liquid in the early morning."
   d. "Eating six smaller meals rather than three large meals will often decrease nausea."

18. Mary asked the nurse if she could drink wine before going to sleep because wine helped her to relax. Which of the following would be the best response?
   a. "A couple of glasses a week would be all right."
   b. "It's best to avoid alcohol in pregnancy because the safe amount is not known."
   c. "Beer is safer to drink than wine."
   d. "Because you're entering your fourth month, it should be all right."

19. Breathing techniques are an important aspect of preparation for labor to prevent ineffective breathing. Which of the following best describes the function of breathing techniques during labor?
    a. Breathing techniques can eliminate pain and will give the expectant parents something to do to occupy their minds.
    b. Breathing techniques reduce the risk of fetal distress by increasing uteroplacental perfusion.
    c. Breathing techniques facilitate relaxation and require concentration, which may reduce the perception of pain.
    d. Breathing techniques can eliminate pain so less analgesia and anesthesia are needed.

20. Mary and John are attending a childbirth class. They asked the nurse, "Why is back massage, especially pressure against the sacral area, soothing to the woman during labor?" Which of the following would be the nurse's best response?
    a. "As the baby descends, there is pressure from inside; the counterpressure from massage eases the discomfort."
    b. "This pressure helps the baby rotate during its passage down the birth canal."
    c. "If the baby is in the posterior position, it helps the baby turn."
    d. "Lying in bed during labor makes the mother's back hurt."

21. The doctor told the nurse that Mary has an android pelvis. The nurse questioned if Mary may need to have a cesarean birth. The doctor would most accurately respond with
    a. "Android is a flat female pelvis."
    b. "Mary has a contracted pelvis so she must be prepared for a cesarean birth."
    c. "Arrest of labor is frequent, thus requiring forceps manipulation or a cesarean birth."
    d. "You tell Mary that there is no

problem; she will have a vaginal delivery."

22. There are several theories for the cause of the onset of labor. The theory that states the need for inhibition of uterine contractility throughout pregnancy is known as the
    a. oxytocin theory
    b. prostaglandin theory
    c. fetal endocrine control theory
    d. progesterone deprivation theory

23. A nurse who examines a patient and finds a transverse lie may conclude which of the following?
    a. This is the woman's first baby.
    b. This woman has had several babies.
    c. This woman has a small uterus.
    d. This woman has pelvic contracture or placenta previa.

24. Which one of the following is *not* a sign of impending labor?
    a. bloody show
    b. rupture of membranes
    c. back pain
    d. patterned and rhythmic contractions

25. What stage of labor is the woman in when she is in the active phase of labor?
    a. stage one
    b. stage two
    c. stage three
    d. stage four

26. A female infant was born vaginally at 7:03 A.M. At 5 minutes, the heart rate is 100 beats per minute, the cry is lusty with active motion of the extremities and a completely pink body. What is the 5-minute Apgar score for this neonate?
    a. 5
    b. 7
    c. 9
    d. 10

27. Following delivery, the infant is placed in the radiant warmer to prevent hypothermia. Your first nursing action is to
    a. Cover the infant with a warm blanket.
    b. Place identification bands on the infant.

226

c. Maintain respiration.

d. Administer vitamin K.

28. To promote drainage of mucus, you place the infant in which of the following positions to prevent ineffective airway clearance?
   a. Sims
   b. Trendelenburg
   c. lithotomy
   d. supine

29. Shortly after delivery, you note that Mary's uterus is one finger below the umbilicus and is displaced to the right of the abdomen. Your first priority would be to
   a. Encourage Mary to void.
   b. Vigorously massage Mary's fundus.
   c. Administer an oxytocic drug.
   d. Administer a tocolytic drug.

30. During the fourth stage of labor, Mary asks, "Why do you keep pressing on my uterus? It sure is sore." You respond
   a. "I need to massage your fundus vigorously to prevent hemorrhage."
   b. "It's important to check your uterus frequently to make sure you don't bleed too much."
   c. "I realize it hurts but it must be done."
   d. "I'm following the doctor's orders."

31. You explain to Mary that right after delivery, the top of the uterus should feel
   a. firm, in the midline, below the umbilicus
   b. firm, to the right of the midline, and above the umbilicus
   c. soft, in the midline, at the umbilicus
   d. soft, to the right of the midline, and above the umbilicus

32. Jan, a 26-year-old primigravida, was admitted to the hospital in the active stage of labor. About 4 hours later, you note that her contractions are not strong enough to cause the cervix to dilate and the uterine tone has decreased. Which of the following would be your nursing diagnosis?

a. High Risk for hypotonic uterine dysfunction related to ineffective contractions
b. High Risk for hypertonic uterine dysfunction related to ineffective contractions
c. High Risk for uterine dysfunction related to contracted pelvis
d. High Risk for uterine dysfunction related to maternal psychosis

33. When planning Jan's care, which of the following interventions would receive the highest priority?
   a. evaluation of blood loss
   b. evaluation of status of membranes
   c. evaluation of maternal and fetal vital signs
   d. evaluation of emotional status

34. Jan's physician ordered oxytocin administration by infusion pump. When monitoring the augmentation of labor, which nursing action would receive the highest priority?
   a. assessment of maternal vital signs
   b. assessment of fetal heart rate
   c. assessment of urinary output
   d. assessment of contractions for frequency, duration, and intensity

35. Kay, a 29-year-old multigravida at 38 weeks' gestation, was admitted to the hospital with painless bright red bleeding and mild contractions every 7 to 10 minutes. While admitting Kay, the nurse will perform all of the following tasks *except*
   a. assessment of maternal vital signs
   b. assessment of fetal heart rate
   c. assessment of contractions
   d. assessment of cervical dilatation

36. Vaginal bleeding during the intrapartal period creates a high-risk situation. Based on Kay's symptoms, which of the following conditions would she most likely have?
   a. abruptio placentae
   b. bloody show
   c. ectopic pregnancy
   d. placenta previa

37. To determine fetal status during Kay's

labor, the nurse will assess fetal heart rate with a

a. stethoscope
b. fetoscope
c. external monitor
d. internal monitor

38. When caring for Kay during labor, the nurse should be particularly alert for
a. decreased urinary output
b. anxiety and fatigue
c. discomfort with contractions
d. hemorrhage

39. Kay's physician told her that she has a complete placenta previa and will need to have a cesarean birth. Kay becomes wide-eyed and begins to cry; she asks, "Why do I need to have a cesarean?" Which one of the following would be your best response to prevent the potential for knowledge deficit?
a. "Ask your physician when he returns."
b. "You need a cesarean to prevent hemorrhage."
c. "The placenta is covering 75% of the internal cervical os and the fetus cannot be delivered vaginally."
d. "The placenta is completely covering the opening of the uterus, so the baby cannot be delivered through the vagina."

40. A transverse lie is when the fetus is positioned in a horizontal rather than vertical plane. Which of the following could be the reason for this position?
a. placenta previa
b. abruptio placentae
c. posterior fundal placenta attachment
d. anterior fundal placenta attachment

41. If the patient has been in true labor for 12 hours and she has been diagnosed as having borderline pelvic measurements, the nurse should prepare the patient for which one of the following procedures?
a. ultrasonography
b. cesarean delivery
c. radiographic pelvimetry
d. manual internal pelvic measurement

42. Dalene is a 42-year-old primipara who is both excited and concerned about her pregnancy. She and her husband delayed pregnancy until their careers were established; then, when she wanted to get pregnant, it took over 2 years. Dalene is a candidate for prenatal diagnosis because of her age. Amniocentesis for prenatal diagnosis of genetic defects is usually done during which period of gestation?
a. 8 to 10 weeks' gestation
b. 14 to 16 weeks' gestation
c. 26 to 28 weeks' gestation
d. 32 to 34 weeks' gestation

43. Baby Girl Loveland is delivered by cesarean section. Her mother is diabetic who has experienced "good control" for 6 years prior to and during pregnancy. The baby is being cared for by the LDRP primary nurse who is also caring for her mother. The plan for care of this infant should include assessments for which of the following conditions?
a. jaundice, hydrocephalus, and seizures
b. LGA, inability to maintain body temperature, and enlarged brain
c. congenital anomalies, hemangioma, and mongolian spots
d. excessive weight, respiratory distress, and tremors

44. Marsha, age 19, was diagnosed as having diabetes mellitus when she was 12 years old. She is in her 36th week of pregnancy. Her insulin and diet have been closely regulated throughout her pregnancy. The physician orders a number of tests to measure fetal well-being. In comparing the results with previous ones, which of the following would the nurse report to the physician immediately?
a. decreased urine estriol
b. decreased bilirubin
c. increased creatinine
d. increased L/S ratio

45. Marsha has progressed through her pregnancy well. At 36 weeks' gestation,

following several tests of fetal well-being, her primary care provider decides she should be induced early. Why would this *not* be considered unusual intervention in this instance?

a. The pregnant diabetic at term tends to be at increased risk for infection.
b. If allowed to go to term, the diabetic infant tends to be large, leading to cephalopelvic disproportion.
c. The risk of severe hypoglycemic crisis during labor increases for the pregnant diabetic when she is near term.
d. The placenta of a diabetic mother tends to degenerate early, causing fetal distress.

46. Gloria Lane, a 32-year-old multipara, had a cesarean delivery at 39 weeks' gestation secondary to an active herpes virus type II infection. The amniocentesis done at 38 weeks' gestation was negative for herpes virus antibodies; however, Mrs. Lane had pustular lesions on her vulva. In preparing Mrs. Lane for discharge, which of the following should the nurse include?

a. the proper way to provide fundal massage for a relaxed uterus
b. proper technique for scrubbing hands and gowning
c. the importance of bed rest for 1 week in order to avoid fatigue
d. the necessity of having someone else care for the infant until after her 6-week postpartum check-up

47. Most elevated temperatures that occur in the first 24 hours postpartum are due to which one of the following?

a. dehydration due to diuresis
b. breast engorgement
c. vaginal infection
d. uterine infection

48. If a newly delivered woman has been in labor for 30 hours and the membranes have been ruptured for 24 hours, which of the following complications would the nurse want to be aware that may occur?

a. endometritis
b. endometriosis
c. salpingitis
d. pelvic thrombophlebitis

49. Which one of the following conditions would alert the nurse to a possible postpartum hemorrhage?

a. long labor (16 hours) and delivery of twins
b. cesarean birth
c. premature delivery
d. precipitous labor and delivery

50. A postpartum psychosis is a rare phenomenon but does occur. Which one of the following behaviors would alert the nurse to the possibility of this occurrence?

a. displaying great excitement over the birth experience
b. crying spells in the early postpartum period
c. complaints of fatigue and therefore not wanting to care for baby
d. asking for pain medication and complaining of pain more than usual

51. A 17-year-old primigravida delivered a 6-lb, 8 oz girl 8 hours ago. In assessing this patient, which of the following assessments would require nursing intervention?

a. temperature of 100.2°F (37.9°C)
b. pulse rate of 60 beats per minute
c. perineal pad soaked with clots every 20 minutes
d. excessive urination

52. If the fundus is above the umbilicus and shifts to one side, what should be the nursing diagnosis?

a. Check first for a full bladder.
b. Massage the uterus.
c. Suspect retained placental fragments.
d. Suspect clots in the uterus.

53. An infant born to a narcotic-addicted mother may exhibit all except which one of the following behaviors?

a. poor feeding
b. tremors
c. high-pitched cry

d. decreased reflex irritability

54. Characteristics of the infant with fetal alcohol syndrome include which one of the following?
    a. a large head
    b. shorter length than usual for a term infant
    c. a smaller sized body and head
    d. heart defects

55. The nurse notices that a newborn is becoming jaundiced 12 hours after birth. Which would be the best nursing action?
    a. Reassure the mother that this is physiological jaundice and normal.
    b. This is not normal physiological jaundice and bilirubin blood levels should be assessed.
    c. The mother is breast-feeding, and this is normal.
    d. Alert the mother that the infant may need an exchange transfusion.

56. Jane, a 20-year-old gravida 2 para 1 at 18 weeks' gestation, is seen in the prenatal clinic for her second visit. Assessment reveals FHR 144 with Doptone, no edema, urine protein negative, weight 124 lb, blood pressure 112/72, temperature 98°F, pulse 84, respirations 18; VDRL negative, hemoglobin 10 g/dL, hematocrit 32%. Jane states, "I've been extremely tired and have had several dizzy spells." The nurse's best response would be:
    a. "Tiredness and dizziness are normal during early pregnancy."
    b. "Your laboratory findings and vital signs are within the normal range."
    c. "Your hemoglobin is low, which could cause these symptoms."
    d. "You are developing preeclampsia."

57. Betty, a 24-year-old gravida 1 para 0 insulin-dependent diabetic, is seen in the clinic at 24 weeks' gestation. She stated that the doctor told her that due to her diabetes her baby is at risk. Betty asks, "What does this mean?" The nurse should respond
    a. "The baby will not grow properly and is likely to be small."
    b. "The baby will probably be a diabetic."
    c. "Ask your doctor what he meant."
    d. "There is a possibility that you will go into labor early."

58. Betty asks, "Will my insulin dosage be the same while I'm pregnant?" The nurse should respond
    a. "No, there will be a need for more insulin as your pregnancy progresses."
    b. "Yes, pregnancy does not have an affect on the amount of insulin needed."
    c. "You don't need to be concerned about that."
    d. "Insulin dosage will change, and you'll need to take your insulin every 4 hours."

59. Michelle has a Class II cardiac disease due to rheumatic fever. You discuss the signs of congestive heart failure with her. You know that she understands the danger signals if she indicates that she would report
    a. pigmentation change
    b. frequent cough
    c. tiredness
    d. colostrum

60. Michelle asks, "When will I most likely develop heart problems during my pregnancy?" The nurse should respond that signs of cardiac complications generally become apparent at
    a. 14 to 18 weeks' gestation
    b. 20 to 24 weeks' gestation
    c. 28 to 32 weeks' gestation
    d. 36 to 40 weeks' gestation

61. Helen, a 32-year-old gravida 4 para 2 at 37 weeks' gestation, was admitted to the delivery suite with the diagnosis of abruptio placenta. With this complication of pregnancy, blood loss is
    a. never present
    b. minimal
    c. greater than observed
    d. less than observed

62. The nurse notes the physician's orders for Helen. Which one of the following orders will be of high priority?

a. Type and cross-match for whole blood.
b. Assess maternal vital signs.
c. Assess FHR.
d. Measure fundal height.

63. The major reason for a 3-week proscription for resumption of sexual intercourse is to prevent
a. tearing of the episiotomy
b. vaginal and cervical infection
c. bladder infection
d. dyspareunia

64. A 35-year-old woman who delivered her third child and smokes one pack of cigarettes per day will probably be advised to choose which of the following contraceptive methods?
a. sponge
b. birth control pills
c. sterilization
d. IUD

65. For a woman using a diaphragm for contraception, the nurse should advise her to leave it in place against the vagina for how long after intercourse?
a. 1 hour
b. 12 hours
c. 28 hours
d. 6 hours

66. The same diaphragm can be used indefinitely if it has the proper care and maintains its original quality. Which of the following situations would warrant remeasurement and possibly a refitting?
a. a weight gain or loss of 5 lb
b. surgery involving general anesthetic
c. surgery involving regional anesthesia
d. pelvic surgery

67. Kyle and Kim have not been able to conceive during the 5 years of their marriage. They have never used contraception. They usually have intercourse three or four times a week and both independently express a high degree of sexual satisfaction. They practice some sexual experimentation with position, time, and location for intercourse, and express particular pleasure with the use of additional lubrication with petroleum jelly. Kyle's sperm count is lower than normal, but other assessment data appear to be well within normal limits. Your recommendation for potentially increasing fertility would include which of the following initially?
a. Reduce frequency of intercourse to be less than once a week.
b. Encourage them to achieve greater consistency in how they perform intercourse.
c. Instruct them to eliminate the additional lubrication.
d. Clarify the validity of the degree of the sexual satisfaction.

68. Introduction of radiopaque material into the uterus and fallopian tubes to assess tubal patency is which of the following diagnostic procedures?
a. uterotubal insufflation
b. laparoscopy
c. culdoscopy
d. hysterosalpingography

69. Which of the following nursing interventions is *not* appropriate in a client just admitted with vaginal bleeding in the third trimester of pregnancy?
a. careful admission history
b. specific assessment of amount of bleeding
c. vaginal examination to determine progress of cervical dilatation
d. vital signs every 15 minutes

70. Mrs. Adams is brought into the emergency room following a car accident. She is in her third trimester of pregnancy and states she was wearing her seatbelt. She has no external evidence of injury, but she is experiencing extreme abdominal pain. Her abdomen is enlarging and is rigid on palpation. Fetal monitoring indicates acute fetal distress. Mrs. Adams is most likely experiencing which of the following complications?
a. placenta previa
b. abruptio placenta
c. severe abdominal bruising
d. normal labor stimulated by stress

71. The prognosis for fetal survival follow-

ing abruptio placenta is less than 50%. For infants who survive, there is a high degree of morbidity. Knowing this, nursing intervention should focus on which of the following?

a. monitoring maternal physiologic status
b. monitoring maternal and infant physiologic status
c. providing emotional support regarding the imminent delivery of a deceased or defective baby
d. administering a tocolytic agent to arrest labor

72. Andrea, a 25-year-old multigravida, is admitted to the hospital in labor. Following examination, the physician noted on the chart "left anterior face presentation." The nurse explains to the nursing student assigned to Andrea that the landmark used to designate the fetal position in the pelvis is
a. acromion
b. mentum
c. occiput
d. sacrum

73. The student nurse asks, "What is the position of the fetal head in a face presentation?" In response, the nurse would explain that the head is
a. completely flexed
b. completely extended
c. partially extended
d. partially flexed

74. Cindy, a 22-year-old primigravida, was admitted to the labor unit. Upon examination, the nurse detects a breech presentation in the left anterior position. Which landmark is used to designate the position in the pelvis of a breech presentation?
a. acromion
b. mentum
c. occiput
d. sacrum

75. With a left anterior breech presentation, where would the fetal heart rate be most audible?
a. above the maternal umbilicus and to the left of midline

b. above the maternal umbilicus and to the right of midline
c. in the lower left maternal abdominal quadrant
d. in the lower right maternal abdominal quadrant

76. At 10:12 AM, the nurse notes that Cindy's membranes have ruptured, with leakage of greenish-colored fluid. What substance would account for this color?
a. blood
b. meconium
c. hydramnios
d. caput

77. With a breech presentation, the nurse must be particularly alert for which of the following?
a. quickening
b. ophthalmia neonatorum
c. pica
d. prolapsed umbilical cord

78. Following rupture of membranes, fetal distress in a vertex presentation may be indicated by which of the following?
a. bloody show
b. hydramnios
c. oligohydramnios
d. meconium

79. In the situation outlined in the preceding question, which of the following interventions would receive the highest priority?
a. Assess FHR
b. Call the physician.
c. Assess maternal vital signs.
d. Assess maternal emotional status.

80. A male infant was born at 1:10 PM. The Apgar score was taken at 1 minute and again at 5 minutes. Which of the following 1-minute and 5-minute Apgar scores would indicate the infant is making an appropriate transition to extrauterine life?
a. 1-minute, 2; 5-minute, 5
b. 1-minute, 4; 5-minute, 6
c. 1-minute, 5; 5-minute, 7
d. 1-minute, 8; 5-minute, 9

81. The newborn can increase body heat by all of the following mechanisms *except*

a. crying vigorously
b. shivering like an adult
c. metabolizing brown fat
d. increasing metabolic rate

82. During physical assessment of a newborn, which of the following comparative measurements would necessitate additional investigation?
    a. head circumference 34 cm; chest circumference 31 cm
    b. head circumference 31 cm; chest circumference 33 cm
    c. head circumference 34.5 cm; chest circumference 32 cm
    d. head circumference 32 cm; chest circumference 30 cm

83. Cold stress is harmful to a newborn because of which of the following outcomes?
    a. peripheral vasodilation
    b. alkalosis
    c. decreased metabolic activity
    d. acidosis

84. Nonshivering thermogenesis is a means of increasing body temperature through
    a. increased muscle activity
    b. metabolism of subcutaneous fat
    c. increased metabolic activity
    d. metabolism of brown fat

85. An infant weighing 3000 g, feeding every 4 hours, needs 120 calories/kg of body weight every 24 hours for proper growth and development. How many ounces of 20 cal/oz formula should this infant receive at each feeding in order to meet nutritional needs?
    a. 2 oz
    b. 3 oz
    c. 4 oz
    d. 6 oz

86. Joanna has been diagnosed with acquired immune deficiency syndrome (AIDS) for some time. She has just delivered a preterm infant, 4.5 lb at birth with a large forehead, oblique eyes, and a flattened bridge of the nose. Which of the following priority nursing interventions will need to be planned immediately regarding this infant?

a. Report the birth of an infected infant to the Centers for Disease Control (CDC) in Atlanta as part of your accountability and documentation.
b. Protect the infant from ineffective thermoregulation and impaired gas exchange.
c. Support the mother and her partner as they deal with the crisis of both the mother and newborn having AIDS.
d. Monitor the immunoglobulin and serum antibodies to determine severity of infection and antibody reserves.

87. Baby John experienced a difficult vaginal birth, resulting in a simple linear skull fracture and bruising. His parents are quite alarmed at his appearance and about potential brain damage. Which of the following is accurate information that would guide both care of the infant and support of the parents?
    a. Skull fractures resulting from traumatic birth almost always result in seizure activity and brain damage.
    b. Simple linear skull fractures are usually benign and heal without treatment.
    c. Simple linear skull fractures often result in tears in the meninges, hemorrhage, and brain damage.
    d. Simple linear skull fractures are always benign and do not require special observations or parental support.

88. Phototherapy has been initiated for the Jones baby to treat hyperbilirubinemia. Which of the following nursing interventions would be inappropriate and could cause injury to the infant?
    a. Place the nude infant in the isolette 18 inches from the phototherapy light.
    b. Turn the infant every 2 hours.
    c. Rub an oil-based lotion on infant's skin to prevent drying and cracking.
    d. Cover the infant's eyes with protective patches.

89. Kelly and Kate are newborn twins born

yesterday to Mary and Tim Brown. Mary had a difficult pregnancy and labor, but she and Tim remained excited to share their life with twins. The twins were born shortly before their EDC with adequate birth weight of 2500 g and 2505 g, respectively. Kelly, however, has an undeveloped right hand with a small thumb and forefinger, but only little skin flaps for the other three fingers. Tim cried and wanted to hold Kelly as soon as possible, along with Kate, but Mary refuses to talk about the anomaly and will not look at Kelly's hand or ask to hold her. Mary's reaction could be analyzed as which of the following?

a. a normal grief reaction of denial
b. an unnaturally strong preference for one twin over the other
c. an unhealthy avoidance of dealing with the reality of Kelly's pathology
d. a pathological psychological reaction that will greatly interfere with bonding

90. Methergine (methylergonovine) 2 mg IM is ordered for Dana Young, a 23-year-old primipara 3 hours postdelivery who is experiencing postpartum bleeding. The nurse would be well advised to observe for potential side effects of the drug. They include which of the following?

a. water intoxication
b. sudden hypertension
c. severe hypoglycemia
d. uterine rupture

91. Jerri Lynn is admitted to the postpartum unit with a MgSO4 continuous drip for pregnancy-induced hypertension. Assessment for signs of eclampsia is necessary for at least how many hours postpartum?

a. 6 hours
b. 12 hours
c. 24 hours
d. 48 hours

92. Within a few minutes following delivery of a 6-lb baby boy with Apgars of 4 and 10, Linda complains of severe chest pain. Her respirations are shallow, ranging between 24 and 30 per minute. A pulmonary embolism is diagnosed by lung scan. Linda is placed on heparin sodium IV therapy with periodic coagulation studies. Of the following common postpartum medication orders, which would be contraindicated by the heparin therapy?

a. Colace
b. Parlodel
c. Motrin
d. Tylenol

93. Beth Ann phones the LDRP unit 6 days following delivery of a 9-lb girl infant to ask her primary nurse if she should report her symptoms to her physician. The nurse explores her concerns and advises Beth Ann to call her physician immediately. Of the following complex symptoms, which one would lead the LDRP nurse to advise Beth Ann to call her physician?

a. scant lochia serosa, fatigue, breast tenderness
b. scant lochia serosa, fatigue, perianal soreness
c. scant lochia rubra, temperature >101°F, uterine tenderness
d. scant lochia alba, scant, fatigue, painful hemorrhoids

94. Following cesarean delivery, Mrs. Lane complains of vulvar pain in the area of herpes lesions. Which comfort measure would be most advisable for the nurse to implement?

a. Encourage her to ambulate several times daily.
b. Suggest she wear tampons rather than maternity pads.
c. Apply warm, moist compresses to the vulva several times daily.
d. Administer sitz baths twice daily; change maternity pads frequently.

95. The nurse's first responsibility in the management of postpartum hemorrhage is to do which of the following?

a. Notify the physician prior to taking any action.

b. Massage the uterus firmly until it remains hard.
c. Take the woman's vital signs.
d. Call for blood type and cross-match and have IV equipment ready.

96. Early postpartum hemorrhage is defined as the loss of a certain amount of blood during the first 24 hours following delivery. Which of the following would accurately represent this amount?
a. 100 mL or more
b. 200 mL or more
c. 500 mL or more
d. 600 mL or more

Answer Sheet for Comprehensive Exam

With a pencil, blacken the circle under the option you have chosen for your correct answer.

	A	B	C	D			A	B	C	D			A	B	C	D
1.	○	○	○	○		21.	○	○	○	○		41.	○	○	○	○
2.	○	○	○	○		22.	○	○	○	○		42.	○	○	○	○
3.	○	○	○	○		23.	○	○	○	○		43.	○	○	○	○
4.	○	○	○	○		24.	○	○	○	○		44.	○	○	○	○
5.	○	○	○	○		25.	○	○	○	○		45.	○	○	○	○
6.	○	○	○	○		26.	○	○	○	○		46.	○	○	○	○
7.	○	○	○	○		27.	○	○	○	○		47.	○	○	○	○
8.	○	○	○	○		28.	○	○	○	○		48.	○	○	○	○
9.	○	○	○	○		29.	○	○	○	○		49.	○	○	○	○
10.	○	○	○	○		30.	○	○	○	○		50.	○	○	○	○
11.	○	○	○	○		31.	○	○	○	○		51.	○	○	○	○
12.	○	○	○	○		32.	○	○	○	○		52.	○	○	○	○
13.	○	○	○	○		33.	○	○	○	○		53.	○	○	○	○
14.	○	○	○	○		34.	○	○	○	○		54.	○	○	○	○
15.	○	○	○	○		35.	○	○	○	○		55.	○	○	○	○
16.	○	○	○	○		36.	○	○	○	○		56.	○	○	○	○
17.	○	○	○	○		37.	○	○	○	○		57.	○	○	○	○
18.	○	○	○	○		38.	○	○	○	○		58.	○	○	○	○
19.	○	○	○	○		39.	○	○	○	○		59.	○	○	○	○
20.	○	○	○	○		40.	○	○	○	○		60.	○	○	○	○

Answer Sheet for Comprehensive Exam

	A	B	C	D		A	B	C	D		A	B	C	D
61.	○	○	○	○	73.	○	○	○	○	85.	○	○	○	○
62.	○	○	○	○	74.	○	○	○	○	86.	○	○	○	○
63.	○	○	○	○	75.	○	○	○	○	87.	○	○	○	○
64.	○	○	○	○	76.	○	○	○	○	88.	○	○	○	○
65.	○	○	○	○	77.	○	○	○	○	89.	○	○	○	○
66.	○	○	○	○	78.	○	○	○	○	90.	○	○	○	○
67.	○	○	○	○	79.	○	○	○	○	91.	○	○	○	○
68.	○	○	○	○	80.	○	○	○	○	92.	○	○	○	○
69.	○	○	○	○	81.	○	○	○	○	93.	○	○	○	○
70.	○	○	○	○	82.	○	○	○	○	94.	○	○	○	○
71.	○	○	○	○	83.	○	○	○	○	95.	○	○	○	○
72.	○	○	○	○	84.	○	○	○	○	96.	○	○	○	○

COMPREHENSIVE TEST—ANSWER KEY

1. *Correct response: a*
Bartholin's glands are the glands on either side of the vaginal orifice.
b. The clitoris is female erectile tissue.
c. The parotid gland opens into the mouth.
d. Skene's glands open into the posterior wall of the female urinary meatus.
Analysis/Physiologic/Analysis (DX)

2. *Correct response: b*
Labia majora are raised longitudinal folds of adipose tissue.
a. Labia minora are soft longitudinal folds of skin between the labia majora.
c. The mons pubis is a mound of fatty tissue over the symphysis pubis.
d. The vestibule is the almond-shaped area between the labia minora
Knowledge/Safe care/Assessment

3. *Correct response: d*
A platypelloid pelvis is a flat female pelvis with a transverse oval inlet.
a, b, and c. These describe a gynecoid pelvis, an android pelvis, and an anthropoid pelvis, respectively.
Knowledge/Safe care/Assessment

4. *Correct response: c*
The fundus is the upper rounded portion of the uterus between the fallopian tubes.
a. The corpus is the body of the uterus.
b. The decidua is the mucous lining of the uterus during pregnancy.
d. The isthmus is a uterine structure located above the cervix.
Application/Safe care/Assessment

5. *Correct response: b*
The obstetric conjugate should measure 11 cm.
a, c, and d. These are all incorrect answers.
Analysis/Physiologic/Assessment

6. *Correct response: d*
Secretion of estrogen by the fetal gonad results in differentiation as a female.
a. Increased maternal estrogen secretions occurs in all pregnancies.
b. Maternal androgen secretion remains the same as before pregnancy.
c. Secretion of androgen by the fetal gonad would differentiate a male fetus.
Analysis/Physiologic/Analysis

7. *Correct response: c*
Gravida refers to a pregnant woman; para refers to a woman who has given birth to a viable infant.
a, b, and d. See the definitions of gravida and para above.
Application/Safe care/Analysis

8. *Correct response: a*
Human chorionic gonadotropin (HCG) is measured to confirm diagnosis of pregnancy.
b. This is a hormone produced by the ovary.
c. This is a hormone produced by anterior pituitary first half of the menstrual cycle.
d. This is a hormone produced by corpus luteum and placenta that stimulates proliferation of the endometrium and growth of embryo.
Knowledge/Safe care/Assessment

9. *Correct response: b*
The symptoms that suggest but do not confirm pregnancy.
a. This is not considered categorical change of pregnancy.
c. These changes strongly suggest pregnancy.
d. These changes are diagnostic of pregnancy.
Comprehension/Safe care/Assessment

10. *Correct response: b*
Blue-purple color of cervix and vaginal mucous membrane.

a. Braxton's refers to painless intermittent contractions that begin in the fourth month of pregnancy.
c. Softening of the cervix.
d. Flexibility of body of uterus against cervix.

Knowledge/Safe care/Assessment

11. **Correct response: b**
This is done to relieve pressure on the vena cava.
a. This will relieve pressure on vena cava but may exacerbate feelings of faintness.
c. This will not relieve symptoms; must reduce pressure on the vena cava.
d. Decreasing pressure on vena cava will cause symptoms to subside.

Comprehension/Physiologic/Implementation

12. **Correct response: C**
This will help to reduce the muscle cramps immediately.
a. This may decrease discomfort but will not reduce the cramp in the muscle.
b. This may help to relax the muscle in time, but there is a need for immediate reduction of cramp to relieve discomfort.
d. This will not reduce the cramp in the muscle

Comprehension/Physiologic/Implementation

13. **Correct response: c**
Ballottement refers to passive movement of the unengaged fetus.
a. This is not a contraction, but rather the passive movement of the unengaged fetus.
b. This refers to quickening.
d. This is Piskacek's sign.

Knowledge/Physiologic/Implementation

14. **Correct response: d**
This needs evaluation; it could be an abnormal finding because the upper left outer quadrant is where a great number of cancerous lumps are found.
a, b, and c. These are all normal during pregnancy.

Analysis/Health promotion/Evaluation

15. **Correct response: d**
Normally, most weight gain occurs in the second and third trimesters.
a. Usually 2 to 4 lb are gained in the first trimester.
b. The answer is not wrong, but it is not the best.
c. A steady weight gain is important for fetal well-being.

Application/Safe care/Implementation

16. **Correct response: b**
Ultrasonography can help determine gestational age and the approximate date of delivery.
a. Determining sex can be incorrect, and ultrasonography is not done for this purpose.
c. Unfortunately, this is correct; however, it is not advisable to tell patients this.
d. Later fetal anomalies may be seen, but early fetal anomalies need further testing.

Analysis/Safe care/Implementation

17. **Correct response: a**
This is not appropriate because it can increase sodium content.
b. Regular crackers often have much sodium content.
c. Dry meals often decrease nausea.
d. Keeping the stomach full often decreases nausea.

Analysis/Safe care/Implementation

18. **Correct response: b**
Alcohol consumption during pregnancy is associated with fetal defects; no safe amount of consumption has been established.
a, c, and d. Alcohol should be avoided throughout pregnancy.

Application/Safe care/Implementation

19. **Correct response: c**
The pain threshold is, which can reduce the perception of pain.
a. Pain is not eliminated.
b. It is not the breathing but rather the position that increases the uteroplacental perfusion.

d. Breathing techniques can reduce, but not eliminate, pain.
Analysis/Physiologic/Analysis (Dx)

20. Correct response: a
Counterpressure eases discomfort.
b. The baby rotates because of fetal position and configuration of the pelvis.
c. Only midforceps rotation could turn the baby, and this is not often done.
d. This may contribute to the backache, but it is not the best answer.
Analysis/Physiologic/Planning

21. Correct response: c
Arrest of labor is frequent in women with android pelves.
a. This response would be irrelevant to the situation.
b. A platypelloid pelvis, not an android pelivs, is contracted.
d. It is inappropriate to offer false hope. She may indeed have to have a cesarean delivery.
Analysis/Health promotion/Planning

22. Correct response: d
Progesterone keeps the smooth muscle of the uterus from contracting throughout pregnancy. However, near term, the placenta produces less progesterone, which initiates labor.
a. According to this theory, the uterus is increasingly sensitive to oxytocin as pregnancy advances.
b. According to this theory, near term, lipids trigger steroid action and release precursors that increase prostaglandin synthesis.
c. This theory posits that fetal adrenal glands secrete cortical steroids that trigger onset of labor.
Analysis/Physiologic/Analysis (Dx)

23. Correct response: d
These conditions may lead to a transverse lie.
a and b. These have nothing to do with a transverse lie.
c. The capacity of the uterus is the same for all women unless there is pathology present.
Analysis/Safe care/Assessment

24. Correct response: c
Back pain is common in pregnancy and is not a sign of impending labor.
a, b, and d. These are all signs of impending labor.
Comprehension/Health promotion/Assessment

25. Correct response: a
The active phase is when the cervix dilates from about 3 cm to 10 cm.
b. Stage two begins with complete dilatation of the cervix and ends with delivery of the infant.
c. Stage three begins with delivery of the placenta.
d. Stage four is the period 1 to 4 hours after delivery.
Knowledge/Physiologic/Analysis (Dx)

26. Correct response: d
The initial adjustment of this neonate is good, because the heart rate, respiratory effort, muscle tone, reflex irritability, and color are each given a score of 2.
a, b, and c. The heart rate is 100 or over, the respiratory effort and reflex irritability are good because the infant is crying, muscle tone is good and there is active motion, color is completely pink.
Analysis/Physiologic/Analysis (Dx)

27. Correct response: c
The infant must be suctioned and respirations established to maintain life.
a. Blankets are not used to cover the infant in a radiant warmer because the heat warms the outer surface of objects. Also, one needs to be able to observe the infant's color.
b and d. Although these are important, neither is the first priority.
Application/Physiologic/Planning

28. Correct response: b
To facilitate drainage of mucus, the infant is placed in a supine position with the head slightly lowered.
a. This is the position where baby lies on left side with right knee and thigh drawn up toward the chest.

c. This is the position where the baby lies on back with legs flexed and thighs flexed up to the abdomen.

d. This is the position where client lies on back on a flat surface.

Application/Physiologic/Planning

29. Correct response: a

A distended bladder will elevate and displace the uterus in the abdomen.

b. A displaced uterus is generally an indication of a full bladder. Vigorous massage of the uterus will cause unnecessary discomfort for Mary.

c. Oxytocic drugs are administered only if the uterus becomes baggy and will not contract.

d. Tocolytic drugs are used to relax the uterus and to prevent or stop premature labor.

Application/Safe care/Implementation

30. Correct response: b

The nurse's primary responsibility immediately after delivery is to observe for postpartal hemorrhage.

a. The fundus should not be massaged vigorously, because this will cause discomfort and may overstimulate the uterus.

c and d. These are poor responses, because there is no explanation as to why a procedure is being done.

Comprehension/Physiologic/Planning

31. Correct response: a

Right after delivery the fundus should be in the midline midway between the umbilicus and the symphysis pubis.

b. This would indicate the bladder is full.

c. This would indicate that the uterus has relaxed and blood and clots need to be expressed with gentle massage.

d. This indicates that the bladder is full and that the uterus has relaxed and blood and clots need to be expressed with gentle massage.

Comprehension/Safe care/Planning

32. Correct response: a

With hypotonic dysfunction, uterine con-

tractions decrease in strength, as does the uterine tone. The contractions are not strong enough to produce cervical dilatation.

b. Hypertonic uterine dysfunction produces a uterus that does not relax completely between contractions, and contractions are of poor quality.

c. Dystocia due to variations in the passageway interferes with engagement, descent, and expulsion of the fetus and can also be the cause of hypotonic dysfunction.

d. Dystocia due to the psyche can cause anxiety and fear that will prolong labor.

Analysis/Health promotion/Analysis (Dx)

33. Correct response: c

It is important that maternal and fetal vital signs are monitored closely to determine the physiologic status and well-being of the maternal–fetal unit.

a. This is not an indication of hemorrhage at this time.

b and d. While important, the priority is to evaluate the integrity of the maternal–fetal unit.

Analysis/Safe care/Planning

34. Correct response: d

Oxytocin will augment contractions; therefore, it is essential to evaluate the contractions for frequency, duration, and intensity to watch for overstimulation of the uterus.

a, b, and c. These are important to assess, but they are not the highest priority.

Analysis/Safe care/Planning

35. Correct response: d

A sterile vaginal examination would not be done because it could cause hemorrhage. Until a diagnosis is made, no vaginal examination is indicated.

a. Assessment of maternal vital signs is important to determine maternal physiologic status.

b. Assessment of the fetal heart rate is essential to determine fetal well-being.

c. Assessment of contractions for frequency, duration, and intensity is important in evaluating the progress of labor.

Analysis/Safe care/Implementation

36. *Correct response: d*

The cardinal symptom of placenta previa is painless, bright red vaginal bleeding during the last half of pregnancy.

   a. The cardinal symptom of abruptio placenta is painful, board-like uterus with dark red or no vaginal bleeding.

   b. Bloody show is a pink mucus discharge present after the discharge of the mucous plug. Show is caused by pressure from the fetal presenting part against the cervix, causing rupture of capillaries.

   c. Ectopic pregnancy is a gestation that is implanted in a site other than the uterine cavity.

Application/Safe care/Assessment

37. *Correct response: c*

External monitoring will produce a continuous recording of the fetal heart rate (FHR), and show the fetal response to maternal contractions.

   a. A clear, accurate FHR cannot always be obtained with a stethoscope.

   b. FHR is taken periodically with a fetoscope; a continuous recording is preferred to show continuous fetal response.

   d. An internal monitor is not used during labor, because the placenta is at the internal cervical os.

Comprehension/Safe care/Assessment

38. *Correct response: d*

With cervical dilatation and effacement, the placenta will continue to break away from the site of implantation and cause bleeding.

   a, b, and c. These are important aspects to determine, but not of the highest priority.

Comprehension/Physiologic/Assessment

39. *Correct response: d*

The nurse should explain to Kay what the physician meant by "complete placenta previa" and why the cesarean section is needed.

   a. This is a poor response that would tend to increase the patient's anxiety.

   b. It is true that a cesarean section would help prevent further hemorrhage, but this statement does not explain the reason for the cesarean delivery.

   c. In a complete placenta previa, the total internal cervical os is covered by the placenta.

Application/Safe care/Implementation

40. *Correct response: a*

The placenta is low or covering the cervical os and fetus and may not allow for vertical position.

   b. This is separation of a normally implanted placenta.

   c and d. These are examples of normal attachment.

Analysis/Physiologic/Analysis (Dx)

41. *Correct response: c*

A sonogram will give the most accurate measurement.

   a. This will show soft tissue.

   b. This is not done without further evaluation first.

   d. This is not as accurate as pelvimetry and generally is not done during labor.

Analysis/Safe care/Evaluation

42. *Correct response: b*

At 14 to 16 weeks, the uterus is sufficiently out of the pelvis to remove the needed fluid. Also, the pregnancy is sufficiently early to terminate in the event of a fetal defect.

   a. At 8 to 10 weeks' gestation, amniocentesis is considered risky.

   c and d. After 26 weeks' gestation, termination of pregnancy because of fetal defect is not recommended.

Knowledge/Health promotion/Assessment

43. *Correct response: d*

Typically, infants of diabetic mothers (IDM) are large for gestational age (LGA), but because they are less mature, they are at increased risk for respiratory distress and tremors associated with hypoglycemia.

   a. Enlarged viscera are common to IDM

infants, but not hydrocephalus and jaundice.

b. Because of physiologic immaturity, the large IDM infant may have difficulty maintaining body temperature.

c. Congenital anomalies are common but not hemangioma or mongolian spots.

Knowledge/Health promotion/Planning

44. Correct response: a

Falling levels of urine estriol, which usually rise as pregnancy progresses, are indicative of some interference with fetal well-being.

b, c, and d. These all indicate normal fetal maturity.

Analysis/Safe care/Analysis (Dx)

45. Correct response: d

The same circulatory disorders that affect the small blood vessels of the diabetic also affect the vessels of the placenta, resulting in placental insufficiency and leading to fetal distress.

a. Concurrent infections may increase vulnerability in the term diabetic but really depend on additional data.

b. Although diabetic mothers tend to have large babies and the incidence of CDP is greater for these mothers, the decision on the best time of delivery for the infant is based on other factors.

c. Although true for some, it is not the basis for determining appropriate birth time.

Analysis/Safe care/Planning

46. Correct response: b

These measures are essential for preventing direct transmission of the virus to the infant.

a. The fundus should not be massaged following cesarean delivery.

c. This is not necessary and could lead to thrombophlebitis.

d. Although it would be helpful to have help with household chores, Mrs. Lane needs to feel free to mother her infant herself in order to promote attachment.

Analysis/Safe care/Planning

47. Correct response: a

Postpartum patients should be told to force fluids to prevent this.

b. This occurrence does not usually cause temperature elevation.

c. Vaginal infections are rare unless the woman was prone to them prior to delivery.

d. This is rare.

Analysis/Physiologic/Analysis (Dx)

48. Correct response: a

This is an infection of the uterine lining.

b. This is a complicated endocrine problem that can cause gynecological and infertility problems.

c. This is infection of the tube and may occur if endometritis is not cured.

d. This is clot formation in pelvic vessels.

Analysis/Physiologic/Planning

49. Correct response: a

This would cause weakened muscle because of the long labor and overstretching with twins.

b. A cesarean birth does not cause increased uterine bleeding.

c. A preterm birth does not cause more bleeding.

d. A precipitous labor and delivery does not cause more uterine bleeding.

Analysis/Safe care/Planning

50. Correct response: c

This is the best answer because the woman does not want to care for her baby.

a. This is normal behavior; many women are exhilarated.

b. Due to hormone changes, this is common.

d. This may be because of anxiety or lack of knowledge.

Analysis/Psychosocial/Planning

51. Correct response: c

This indicates a postpartal hemorrhage.

a and b. These are within limits.

d. This is normal after delivery, because the pregnant woman who normally holds fluids rids herself of excess fluids.

Analysis/Safe care/Implementation

52. Correct response: a

This is the first thing to assess.

b. If uterus is firm massage is not necessary.

c. Retained placenta fragments cause increased bleeding.

d. The uterus may feel soft.

Analysis/Safe care/Analysis (Dx)

53. *Correct response: d*

Infants born to narcotic-addicted mothers have an increase in reflex irritability and often have continuous body movement.

a. They are poor feeders.

b. They have tremors.

c. They have a high-pitched cry.

Analysis/Safe care/Analysis (Dx)

54. *Correct response: c*

They often are smaller.

a. They do not have a larger head.

b. They are not necessarily shorter in length.

d. This is not necessarily true.

Analysis/Physiologic/Analysis (Dx)

55. *Correct response: b*

Bilirubin needs to be monitored.

a. This is too early for physiological jaundice.

c. Breast-fed babies do have more jaundice, but this is too early for physiologic jaundice.

d. One does not want to frighten the parents unnecessarily.

Analysis/Safe care/Analysis (Dx)

56. *Correct response: c*

Anemia limits the amount of oxygen available in the body.

a. Extreme tiredness and dizziness are not normal signs of pregnancy.

b. Hemoglobin and hematocrit reflect anemia.

d. Subjective and objective data do not support development of pre-eclampsia.

Analysis/Physiologic/Analysis (Dx)

57. *Correct response: d*

There is an increased incidence of premature labor and delivery.

a. Infants are often larger due to fetal hyperinsulinism and hyperglycemia.

b. Diabetes is not demonstrated in the fetus or neonate.

c. This type of response will cause more apprehension in the woman.

Comprehension/Psychosocial/Implementation

58. *Correct response: a*

There is a need to increase the dosage of insulin as pregnancy progresses, because there is progressive insulin resistance due to placental insulinase.

b. Progressive insulin resistance results in the need for dosage adjustment during pregnancy.

c. This response would make the patient more apprehensive.

d. Adjustment of insulin dosage and times are individualized to achieve good control.

Analysis/Psychosocial/Implementation

59. *Correct response: b*

Coughing is primary symptom of congestive heart failure.

a. This is a probable change of pregnancy.

c. This is a presumptive change of pregnancy.

d. This is produced by the mammary gland during pregnancy before onset of lactation.

Application/Health promotion/Evaluation

60. *Correct response: c*

Progressive rise in cardiac output reaches its peak at 28 to 32 weeks' gestation because there is a peak increase in blood volume, stroke volume, and heart rate at this time.

a, b, and d. These time frames are incorrect.

Comprehension/Physiologic/Implementation

61. *Correct response: c*

With abruptio placenta, there is frequently concealed hemorrhage; with greater blood loss observed.

a and b. In these conditions, there is blood loss with abruptio placenta because the placenta tears from the uterus and causes bleeding.

d. Concealed hemorrhage produces *more* blood loss than can be observed.

Comprehension/Physiologic/Assessment

62. *Correct response: a*

Blood loss can be great; therefore, blood replacement is needed.

b, c, and d. These are important but not the highest priority.

Comprehension/Health promotion/Planning

63. *Correct response: b*
A woman is at increased risk for vaginal and vervical infection for the first 3 weeks post-delivery.
   a. The episiotomy is usually fairly well healed in the first week.
   c. Infection could move upward from the vagina and cervix, but this is not the best answer.
   d. This may be true, but it is not the best answer.

Analysis/Physiologic/Planning

64. *Correct response: d*
Of those mentioned, it is the most effective except for sterilization, a largely irreversible method of contraception.
   a. The sponge is not very effective for women who have had several children.
   b. Oral contraceptives are not given to older women who smoke because of the possibility of embolism problems.
   c. Sterilization would not be recommended because of its permanency.

Analysis/Safe care/Planning

65. *Correct response: d*
The diaphragm should remain in place 6 hours after each (if applicable) subsequent intercourse.
   a. Sperm will often be alive and able to permeate cervix and impregnate ova.
   b. This is too long for diaphragm placement; a woman is prone to infection.
   c. This is the same rationale as b; however, this is much more serious.

Analysis/Safe care/Implementation

66. *Correct response: d*
This can change the shape or size of pelvic structures, and refitting of the diaphragm may be necessary.
   a. A weight gain or loss of 10 lb or more is the benchmark indicating that refitting may be necessary.
   b and c. Anesthesia does not have any-

thing to do with anatomical changes of the pelvis.

Analysis/Health promotion/Implementation

67. *Correct response: c*
Petroleum jelly and some water-soluble lubricants have been shown to be spermicidal.
   a. Reducing intercourse will not increase the probability of conception.
   b and d. There are not adequate data at this point to support these as factors in this couple's inability to conceive.

Analysis/Safe care/Implementation

68. *Correct response: d*
Hysterosalpingography involves radiologic examination of the uterine cavity, fallopian tubes, and peritubal area.
   a, b, and c. None of these procedures use a radiopaque material.

69. *Correct response: c*
Vaginal examination should not be performed, or damage to fetal blood vessels may occur and hemorrhage might be worsened.
   a, b, and d. Careful admission history, assessment of bleeding, and vital signs are all indicated in this situation.

Knowledge/Safe care/Implementation

70. *Correct response: b*
These assessment data point to abruptio placenta.
   a, c, and d. The assessment data are typical of abruptio placenta and do not support any of the other disorders listed.

Application/Physiologic/Analysis (Dx)

71. *Correct response: b*
Both mother and infant should be monitored carefully to promote survival and to decrease risk of morbidity.
   a. The infant, as well as the mother, should be monitored.
   c. The death or defectiveness of the baby would probably not be a main focus of action unless the baby dies or had a morbid condition.

d. Tocolytics are contraindicated in abruptio placenta.

Application/Safe care/Implementation

72. Correct response: b
The mentum is used as the landmark to determine fetal position in a face presentation.
  a. The acromion is the landmark used for a shoulder presentation
  c. The occiput is the landmark used for a vertex presentation.
  d. The sacrum is the landmark used for a breech presentation.

Comprehension/Physiology/Assessment

73. Correct response: b
With a face presentation, the head is completely extended.
  a. The head is completely flexed in a vertex presentation.
  c and d. Partial extension or flexion can occur in other presentations.

Comprehension/Safe care/Assessment

74. Correct response: d
The sacrum is used as the landmark to designate the position of a breech presentation in the pelvis.
  a. In a shoulder presentation, the acromion process (scapula) is used as the landmark.
  b. The mentum (chin) is the landmark to designate the position of a face presentation.
  c. The occiput is used as the landmark in a vertex presentation.

Comprehension/Physiologic/Assessment

75. Correct response: a
The fetal heart will best be heard from the fetal upper torso and through the fetal back. With the LSA, the fetal upper torso and back face the left upper maternal abdominal wall.
  b, c, and d. These locations are not the best spots to auscultate the fetal head.

Application/Health promotion/Analysis (Dx)

76. Correct response: b
Upon descent into the pelvis, the fetus in a breech presentation will pass meconium due to compression on the intestinal tract.

  a. Greenish amniotic fluid is not an indication of bleeding.
  c. Hydramnios refers to is an excessive amount of amniotic fluid.
  d. Caput is the occiput of the fetal head that is at the vaginal introitus just before delivery of the head.

Analysis/Health promotion/Analysis (Dx)

77. Correct response: d
There is space available between the presenting part and the cervix, through which the cord can slip.
  a. Quickening is the woman's first perception of fetal movements.
  b. Conjunctivitis of the newborn generally results from maternal gonorrhea.
  c. Pica refers to oral intake of nonfood substances, such as cornstarch, dirt, clay, or plaster by a malnourished person, often seen in a child or pregnant woman in need of nutrients to support growth.

Analysis/Safe care/Analysis (Dx)

78. Correct response: d
With fetal distress, there is an increase in the peristaltic movement of the intestines; thus, the fetus will expel meconium.
  a. Bloody show is the pink mucous discharge that is present after discharge of the mucous plug. Show is caused by pressure from the fetal presenting part on the cervix, causing rupture of capillaries.
  b. Hydramnios is an excessive amount of amniotic fluid.
  c. Oligohydramnios is a decreased amount of amniotic fluid, frequently seen with a fetal urinary tract anomaly.

Application/Safe care/Assessment

79. Correct response: a
Meconium-stained amniotic fluid is a sign of fetal distress, and the FHR must be assessed immediately.
  b, c, and d. These are important interventions, but not the highest priority given the risk to the fetus.

Evaluation/Health promotion/Planning

80. Correct response: d

A set of Apgar scores that are between 7 and 9 indicate good initial adjustment of the neonate when the heart rate, respiratory effort, muscle tone, reflex irritability, and color are evaluated.

    a, b, and c. These scores are indicative of a compromised infant; scores below 4 indicate the neonate is severely depressed.

Analysis/Safe care/Assessment

81.   **Correct response: b**
Newborns cannot shiver.

    a, c, and d. Newborns can raise body heat by crying vigorously, by metabolizing brown fat, and by increasing metabolic rate.

Analysis/Physiologic/Evaluation

82.   **Correct response: b**
The head circumference in a normal infant is larger than the chest circumference.

    a, c, and d. These measurements fall within normal limits (the head circumferences are larger than the chest circumferences) and need no further investigation.

Analysis/Safe care/Analysis (Dx)

83.   **Correct response: d**
Cold stress constricts pulmonary vessels and decreases blood flow, causing hypoxia and an increase in ketone bodies. It also increases metabolic rate and, with hypoxia, causes anaerobic glycolysis and metabolic acidosis.

    a. This is a normal occurrence when the infant is cold.

    b. This is the opposite of acidosis.

    c. This increases metabolic activity.

Analysis/Physiologic/Analysis (Dx)

84.   **Correct response: d**
Cold stress stimulates the sympathetic nervous system to release norepinephrine, which causes the metabolism of brown fat.

    a. This occurs with vigorous activity.

    b. This does not occur in newborns.

    c. This occurs in cold stress of the newborn.

Analysis/Physiologic/Analysis (Dx)

85.   **Correct response: b**
Mathematical calculation: (1) 1.3 kg × 120 cal/kg/day = 36 cal/day. (2) 360 cal/day = 6 feedings per day = 60 cal per feeding. (3) 3.60 cal per feeding = 20 cal/oz = 3 oz per feeding.

    a, c, and d. Based on the calculation, these amounts would be incorrect.

Analysis/Health promotion/Planning

86.   **Correct response: b**
Monitoring for and correcting ineffective thermoregulation and impaired gas exchange would be the highest priority for this newborn.

    a, c, and d. Adequate reporting and documentation, parental support, and determination of infection and antibody levels are very important, but infant thermoregulation and gaseous exchange are a priority.

Application/Safe care/Planning

87.   **Correct response: b**
Simple linear skull fractures generally are benign and heal without treatment.

    a, c, and d. Simple linear fractures are usually benign but would still require careful ongoing assessment and parental support. Depressed fractures are more likely to cause meningeal tears and damage to brain tissue.

Comprehension/Physiologic/Analysis (Dx)

88.   **Correct response: c**
Oil-based lotions or ointments should not be used, because they may cause burns when used with phototherapy.

    a, b, and d. These are correct interventions.

Application/Safe care/Implementation

89.   **Correct response: a**
The inability to discuss or look at pathol-

ogy soon after its occurrence is a normal denial and avoidance that is a part of grieving. Mary will need time and nonjudgmental support in dealing with her disappointment, sadness, and anger over Kelly's anomaly.

  b, c, and d. Mary's response is neither unnatural, unhealthy, or pathological; it is a normal grief response.

Analysis/Psychosocial/Analysis (Dx)

90. *Correct response: b*
Hypertension is a potential side effect of Methergine.

  a, c, and d. Water intoxication, severe hypoglycemia, and uterine rupture are not potential side effects of this drug.

Knowledge/Safe care/Planning

91. *Correct response: d*
Eclampsia is a possibility for as long as 48 hours after delivery in the patient with pregnancy-induced hypertension serious enough to be treated with MgSO4.

  a, b, and c. Assessment should be maintained for at least 48 hours postpartum.

Comprehension/Safe care/Application

92. *Correct response: c*
Motrin is contraindicated in patients receiving heparin therapy.

  a, b, and d. Colace, Parlodel, and Tylenol are all considered compatible with heparin.

Analysis/Safe care/Implementation

93. *Correct response: c*

These symptoms suggest postpartum infection and should be explored further.

  a, b, and d. These are all normal concerns 6 days following delivery.

Application/Safe care/Assessment

94. *Correct response: d*
Sitz baths are comforting, and frequent pad changes will help the lesions to dry.

  a. Ambulation will increase discomfort.
  b. Newly delivered patients should not be encouraged to wear tampons because of the risk of infection.
  c. This will keep the lesions moist, when keeping them dry promotes healing.

Comprehension/Physiologic/Planning

95. *Correct response: b*
The primary cause of postpartum hemorrhage is uterine atony. Fundal massage promotes the contraction of the uterus.

  a. Notifying the physician is not necessary before independent nursing interventions.
  c and d. Vital sign monitoring and blood typing and cross-matching may become necessary, but uterine massage is the initial recommended intervention.

Knowledge/Safe care/Implementation

96. *Correct response: c*
By definition, blood loss of 500 mL or more during the first 24 hours following delivery is considered early postpartum hemorrhage.

  a, b, and d. These amounts don't constitute the definition of early postpartum hemorrhage.

Knowledge/Physiologic/Assessment

Index

Page numbers followed by *f* indicate figures; those followed by *t* indicate tabular material.

A

Abdomen, postpartal changes in, 119
Abortion, spontaneous, 158–160
    assessment and, 159
    etiology and pathophysiology of, 158–159
    evaluation and, 160
    nursing diagnoses and, 159
    planning and implementation and, 159–160
Abruptio placenta, 161–162
    assessment and, 162
    etiology and pathophysiology of, 161–162
    evaluation and, 162
    nursing diagnoses and, 162
    planning and implementation and, 162
Adrenal glands, during pregnancy, 63
Amniocentesis, 90
Amnion, 29
Amnioscopy (transcervical fetal visualization), 90
Amniotic fluid (bag of waters), 31
Amniotic membrane, rupture of, 102
    artificial, 171–172
    premature. *See* Premature rupture of membranes
Analgesia, during labor, 107
Anemia, antepartal, 156–157
    assessment and, 156
    etiology and pathophysiology of, 156
    evaluation and, 157
    nursing diagnoses and, 156
    planning and implementation and, 156–157
Anesthesia, during labor, 108
Antepartal care, 83–95
    assessment and, 84–85
      diagnostic tests and procedures and, 85
      health history in, 84–85
      risk factor assessment and, 85, 86t–87t
    assessment in, 90–94
    evaluation and, 95
      fetal well-being and, 85, 87–90
    evaluation of fetal well-being and
      electronic fetal heart monitoring and, 89–90

essential concepts of, 85, 87
    fetal heart rate and, 87
    fetal movements and, 89
    measurement of fundal height and, 88–89
    ultrasonography and, 87–88
  factors affecting antepartal experience and, 84
  goals of, 84
  nursing diagnoses and, 93–94
  nursing management and, 90–95
  nursing responsibilities and, 84
  planning and implementation and, 94–95
Antepartal complications, 153–165
    abruptio previa, 161–162
    anemia, 156–157
    ectopic pregnancy, 162–163
    essential concepts of, 154
    hemolytic disease of fetus and newborn, 157–158
    hyperemesis gravidarum, 155–156
    nursing management of at-risk patients and, 154–155
    placenta previa, 160–161
    pregnancy induced hypertension, 163–165
    spontaneous abortion, 158–160
Anticipatory stage of childrearing, 65
Areola, 16
Artificial rupture of membranes (AROM), 171–172
Asphyxia. *See* Birth asphyxia
Assessment, 6, 6t
Autosomal dominant inheritance, 32
Autosomal recessive inheritance, 32

B

Bag of waters (amniotic fluid), 31
Barbiturates, during labor, 107
Bartholin's (vulvovaginal) glands, 15
Basal body temperature (BBT)
    contraception and, 51
    in infertility, 41–42

249